A King's Buffe
Hidden Treasures

PREFACE 4

ACHIEVE A DIFFERENT MINDSET 6

ABOUT CARB COUNTING 8

THE BATTLE 9

A LITTLE BIT ABOUT THE AUTHOR 15

LET'S START OUT IN THE COTTAGE HOUSE PANTRY 20

MUSTARDS 21
HERBAL OILS 30
COTTAGE HOUSE DAIRY 37
GETTING TO KNOW YOUR CHEESES 51

LESSONS FROM THE COTTAGE HOUSE 55

HERE ARE A FEW TIPS: 56

MORE FROM THE COTTAGE HOUSE 57

ON TO THE SAUCES 61
ON TO THE DIPS 67

READY FOR APPETIZERS 90

ABOUT BREAKFAST 118

LET'S TALK ABOUT OMELETS A LITTLE BIT 122

DINNER SELECTIONS 146

DESERTS 211

A TIME TO REFLECT 233

GIVING THANKS 236

Dedicated to;

My wonderful Husband Mike, for his encouragement and support.

Jan, my earthly angel, just for putting up with me for twenty two years.

Darlene, my spiritual counter-part, who's been on that long, strange chubby journey with me and can still laugh about it after twenty some years.

William Joseph Wilson, who faithfully and unselfishly gave many long hours of his time to this project.

The family that I am extremely fortunate to have around me. I would like to acknowledge everyone individually, but that would be another whole book. Thank you Mom and Dad!

And above all, endless Praise to my Heavenly Father, who without His splendid Grace, I could not be or do anything at all!

In Memory of Robert C. Atkins, M.D.

A true pioneer who led the way for millions of people to overcome obesity as well as other health related problems. Thank you for your many years of commitment and sacrifice. Thank you for your relentless dedication to overcoming adversity. You have changed the lives of multitudes of people and your work will always live on. You are a true Hero to the cause! May God Bless You!

PREFACE

*T*o all of my friends out there who can not get past the carbohydrate addiction. The addiction is real. It is not going to go away and hopefully together we can learn how to live with it and enjoy every bite of food that we eat and yet manage our lifestyle at the same time.

We feel that the very reason low-carb eating plans are unsuccessful for any length of time, is that most recipes do not offer you enough decadence to make you want to trade in your high-carb calories, to make the switch for the long haul.

Our mission at the Cottage House is to offer you recipes that are so rich, so tasty and satisfying that you will be willing to make some changes that will last you a life time. As the saying goes, "Give a man a fish and he can eat for a day, teach a man to fish and he can eat for a lifetime!" Our hope is that you can walk away from this book having learned something about those changes. The only thing you have to lose are those dreaded extra pounds!

We all know what the low-carb eating plan is. The real problem lies in finding a way to eliminate the challenges that cause our best efforts to de-rail time and time again.

The Cottage House has created this book from necessity, for all of our carb-junkie friends out there who need help staying on track.

Searching endlessly for low-carb recipes that I could actually live with over the long haul... I pretty much struck a zero. These recipes just weren't good enough to make me want to trade in my potatoes, popcorn and pasta! We know as carb-junkies, food pretty much has to be over the edge in flavor and richness or we are really not that interested now, are we?

By request, I will share with you some of the "Hidden Treasures of the Cottage House". Recipes created for carb-junkies by carb-junkies who know the value of an opulent meal or a richly satisfying snack. Someone who suffers as you do. Someone who understands you, not someone who has never been more than fifteen pounds over goal weight in their life. We are in this together!

Life is a celebration! It is not just about food. It's about living, loving, sharing and caring. It's about being good to ourselves and others, especially now in these times of uncertainty.

Come along with me on a Cottage House adventure as we explore not only fabulous recipes, but a variety of little insights on how to relax, share with friends, tips on cooking, little pearls of wisdom, little celebrations of life and even a little spiritual meditation. This is what life is all about. Let's celebrate!

Before we embark on our adventure, let's relax a little and create a bit of a different atmosphere. At this time, we may want to clear out some of the day's anxieties. Sit down in a comfortable place, take a few deep breaths and exhale slowly. Here we go!

ACHIEVE A DIFFERENT MINDSET

To achieve a different mind set, come along with me to another place and time where life is peaceful, romantic and quiet. Imagine an English garden with the fragrance of wild flowers permeating the air. Maybe it's the Heather or Foxglove that soothes your soul. The air seems crisp and fresh. You notice the hummingbirds dancing freely around you as though they were floating in the air. Perhaps a stroll down the path helps you realize the absolute beauty of this garden. Maybe you would like to sit on that comfortable bench near the stream and listen to it quietly trickle by. You notice the sun glistening softly off the top of the water. Oh! How beautiful this is! A fawn, sipping water has been alerted by your presence. She looks at you almost as if she trusts you completely and goes about her way.

The birds are chirping and by now, the sun is nestling ever so slowly into the horizon, enough so that the lamps along the pathway light up to a soft warm glow. Perhaps you are sipping a cup of minted tea. Take a few deep breaths and exhale slowly. Take it all in. Maybe you can't remember the last time you felt this relaxed. Isn't this wonderful? Would you like to come here again?

Come here again or create your own place. Custom made just for you. A place that is yours and yours alone. A place that can be anything you want it to be. A place you can go to get away from the day's anxieties for a while. See how soon they seem to fade away. Go there and go there often. Sip a cup of tea or a glass of wine while you are there. Be good to yourself. You deserve it!

Life is too short. Stop and smell the roses. God has given you a sunset to relax to after a hard days work. He has given you stars and a moon to fall asleep to at night... Sunshine to smile at you, as you wake in the morning. He has sent you flowers everywhere if you just take the time to look. Do we get so busy in life that we miss all the gifts that are right in front of us to enjoy? If we slow down long enough to open our eyes we may see them... a smile, a kind word, a show of help, a touch of compassion, a hug from a friend. All free for the taking and free for the giving! This is what life is all about isn't it? Happy giving!

Now, go to your quiet place and relax. Light some candles, soak in the tub, read a good book, but whatever you do...ESCAPE! Escape the rigors of the day. Take a load off. Your mind will be happy, your body will be happy and your soul will be happy! Everybody needs a break. Be good to yourself and others and the world will be a much better place indeed!

ABOUT CARB COUNTING

Although many recipes in this book are no carb recipes, there are some that do contain minimal carbs. If you are seriously restricting carbohydrates and view a recipe that seems "questionable" to you, it would be in your best interest to purchase a "carb-counter" book available in most book stores, so that you can make your own choices.

The recipes in this book are intended to be used as "alternatives" to high carb foods. Remember, we are trying to find recipes we can live with for the long haul.

When it comes to looking at the recipes, for example, the Bananas Foster...if you would like to eat it but you say to yourself, I can't do that...there's 26 carbs just in the banana, if the Gelato and the sugar free caramel sauce do not have any carbs, then just eat two or three small pieces of banana on top of your Gelato to get the flavor and you will have minimal carbs. No one said you have to eat the whole banana. The same is true for the salsa's or whatever else has minimal carbs. A little dab will do ya! We are going for quality not quantity. We are trying to maximize the flavor, not the food. If your objective happens to be "more" food on a particular day, make sure it is more of the no carb food.

The "idea" of this book is to help you get the "most" out of your eating experience all the way around. This is what will help keep you on track. To get the "most" out of anything in life, you have to have some FUN doing it or you probably won't do it. So, let's make up our mind to have some FUN and let's just do it! Let's have a blast!

I personally do not advocate total carb restriction when it comes to fruits and vegetables. The good Lord put them here for a reason. I've never seen anyone obese from eating too many of them, they are not addictive and life is too short!

THE BATTLE

Friends, if you are like me and a million other people out there, you know the pain of a carb-junkie. We are in a class all of our own. We can run but we can't hide. Those carbs keep coming at us. They are going to find us and consume us, like it or not! As long as we keep eating them, they are going to give us the extra baggage we all dread. I know. I've tried it all. It may not be fair, but it is a fact!

This is not a medical book, nor does it make any claims as such. There are a hundred books on the market written by reputable physicians to which you can refer, who can explain to you why, if you are a carb-junkie and continue to eat those carbs, it's almost impossible to lose weight. As always, you should check with your regular physician before embarking on any health related changes.

If you do not know how to determine whether or not you are a carb-junkie, here is a basic quiz. In fact, let's call it the "carb-junkie quiz".

- At a typical breakfast, can you eat the meat and eggs without the toast and hash browns?
- Can you eat the meat and vegetables at dinner without the potatoes rice or pasta?
- Do you eat the potato, rice or pasta first at your meal, moving on the meat and vegetable if you still have room?

or...

- Do you eat the meat and vegetable first and then go to the potato, rice or pasta if you still have room? Interesting question?
- Do you wake up in the morning craving sweets?
- At a party, do you hit the chips and dip like a northern while speeding right past the veggies and low-carb dip?

- Do you find that the more you eat sugars and starches, the more you crave them?
- Have you ever secretly eaten the whole cake, little by little, hoping that no one would know it was you? Or, all at once?
- Are you really angry because some people can eat it all and never gain a pound, but all you have to do is look at food and gain weight?

I don't think I have to tell you that if you answered yes to one or more of these questions, this book should stay in your hands. Because my friend, there is help on the way! You are with friends and together, we are going to succeed!

Let's talk about "us" for a moment. What makes "us" different from the "other group" of people? (We can say "other group" because that's how isolated we feel sometimes, don't we?). If you want to add a little humor here, let's call them the "spandex crowd". You know who they are! They are the ones who would rather go out and run a 10K than sit home, rent a good movie and pop some popcorn! It's the guy who's been at the gym all day, on his day off, slamming down bottled water, not the guy who's been out in the garage all day slamming down brewski's. I'm sure that we can call them the "spandex crowd" without insulting them, because you can bet your bottom dollar they would not want to trade places with us by any stretch of the imagination. And of course, can we blame them? Take your compliment "spandex crowd".

Girlfriends... it's your best friend. The one who can do lunch with you and order a Caesar salad and an iced tea while you order the half pound cheeseburger, with bacon, fries AND a coke, while you are telling her that you might as well eat it because that is all you will be eating for the day. Right! Like she believes you? It could happen!

Don't you hate the friend who orders a bowl of vegetable soup for lunch and passes on the bread saying, "No thanks! I couldn't eat another bite?" What orbit is she FROM, you ask yourself. "I'll show her! I'm no different than her! I'll order the soup only, just like her! I can always pick up a burger on the way home after I drop her off anyway." Doesn't sound like anyone you know does it? If it doesn't... Good for you. I mean that. Really!

What makes us say, "There's no way I can eat the steak without the potato?" Or simply, "I just can not live without my chocolate!" I'll tell you friends, the answer is simple. We are addicted to carbohydrates. It isn't fair, but it is a fact! Try living without them and see who's kidding!

Are we now ready to admit that we are carb-junkies? No? Still not convinced that this is you we are talking about? Please remain seated! Have you ever over-dosed on a green salad? How about fish, turkey, pork or beef? Scrambled eggs, carrots, celery, onions or broccoli? I don't think that there is a part of over-dose that applies here right? Now, let me ask you the next question. Have you ever over-dosed on chocolate desert? Potato chips, cookies or pizza? Better yet, how about a fried chicken dinner with all the fixin's? And the wing dinger, the big turkey dinner? Is the *FOG* lifting yet? When was the last time you got up in the middle of the night, snuck out to the fridge and stole a handful of broccoli? I think maybe it was that big fat piece of chocolate cake sitting next to the broccoli myself! Can you imagine the taste of broccoli in your tooth paste "night mouth" come morning? But that chocolate cake just somehow mixes with that minty toothpaste! I don't see a problem here! Slides right down!

Now that we have realized that we have a little problem here, and we *SHOULD* be realizing it, let's address some of the stumbling blocks that seem to get in the way of our progress all the time. It's because of who we are! We are carb-junkies! Like we said before, we are in a class all our own.

Boarding a 10 speed bike and riding it 50 miles... or 10... or 3? That's just not happening for most of us! Fair enough? Getting into physical fitness? That usually constitutes walking down to the gas station for exercise, picking up a chocolate glazed doughnut, and hoping to wear it off by the time we get home. But, that nice neighbor drives by and offers us a lift. There we are, home in 30 seconds. Maybe not, maybe we walked all the way... It could happen! Do you like this excuse? "Frankly, I just don't have the time or the energy to do it". That one is a classic for carb-junkies and we say it with authority, because if anyone knew how hard we worked all day, they would understand why we are too tired, right? (Could it be that padded office chair that gave us such a work-out today?).

To be real honest, the biggest amount of exercise I ever got at work was when they moved the vending machine to a different hallway.

What if I told you that while exercise is great for your health, mind and body and of course speeds up weight loss, that if you could not bring yourself to do it, it might not be entirely necessary in losing weight? I would never recommend not exercising, but what if I told you that by minimizing carbs you could actually start getting energy that you never knew existed? Do you know why that is? It is the excess carbs that drag us down and steal our energy! Do you believe that what I say to you is true? Let me ask you this question. Have you ever eaten a large green salad with all the goodies and had to go lie down and take a nap after you ate it? I can actually say, that has never happened to me. Now, have you ever eaten a big turkey dinner with all the fixin's and had to go lay down and take a nap after you ate it? Blame it on the Tryptophan, I call it serious carb overload. You know we have been so lethargic after a dinner like that, we have had to lie down and sleep it off or we would have fallen down! If that meal had a warning label on it, it would read... caution! Do not eat this meal and try to operate a moving vehicle. Operate it? I wouldn't have enough energy to get into it, let alone try to operate it! Still blaming the Tryptophan? I can sit down to the table and eat a 6-8 oz. turkey steak with a few veggies on the side and get up from the table and clean the whole kitchen! About that turkey dinner... how much turkey do you really eat in that turkey dinner any way? Be honest! 3oz. of turkey meat, half a pound of mashed potatoes, half a pound of dressing, a slathering of that good gravy, a quarter pound of those brown sugar, marsh-mellowed sweet potatoes and at least a now and later piece of that praline pumpkin or pecan pie, with ice cream! That is nothing but a carbohydrate infestation! Forget the turkey! The turkey is just an excuse to get to the rest of the meal! I am trying to make a point here... Is it working? Are you starting to see the enemy? Just how much energy are we being robbed of? Maybe if we weren't constantly being robbed, we would have more energy to get up and move. The more we move around, the more we speed up our metabolisms. The more we speed them up, the more weight we lose. The more weight we lose the more we become inspired, and we would be doing all this without really trying. It doesn't get any easier than this! Isn't this amazing?

And last but not least, have you ever had anyone tell you that if you want to be thin, eat like a thin person! Glory Be!! Most thin people can eat far more than us straight-away! Who's not getting this?

Why not start now and try to conquer the little things that add up to the big things? Something we can live with? We can make changes that are a sure thing, and the one thing we carb-junkies have to have is BIG TASTE and BIG SATISFACTION! This is our real enjoyment. We love to eat! Hands down, we are comfort food people and if it isn't tasty and satisfying, it isn't worth eating! Am I right? We always like to feel like we are getting the best, and tasting the best, don't we? We want decadent! We want opulent!

Suppose I ask you this question. If you could have the richness, opulence and taste, and it would taste as good if not better than some of your high-carb foods, would you be willing to replace some of your high-carb food with it? If I could give you a large portion of beef, fish, pork, poultry or seafood with a sauce so decadent that you might even be willing to forget about your potato, would you try it? If it was even better than you thought it could be, would you be willing to try it again? Do you believe that if I could offer you something richer and tastier than the carb you are stuck on, that you would have an easier time letting it go?

If that is the case, I hope this is the place you want to be right now...getting ready for our adventure together!

A LITTLE BIT ABOUT THE AUTHOR

My very first experience in the work-a-day world about thirty years ago was an opportunity to become a trained chef, in "International Cuisine" by the corporation that I was lucky enough to work for and can you believe it was a requirement of the job? Was that a golden opportunity or what? Trained to use the finest of ingredients, the richest of creams, the tastiest of butters, the best olive oil and the most decadent of chocolates! To round out my early career, I decided to apprentice in a bakery to develop my skills in bakery or pastry as it is called today! Combine all that with a LARGE PASSION for cooking and baking and what do you have? A chef with a sluggish metabolism and a lethal dose of extra baggage accumulated over the years! I've heard it said once or twice... Never trust a skinny chef. Did I have to take that so literally?

Let me be personal with you for a moment. Have you ever, just for a moment, felt sorry for yourself? If you have, I want you to know, you are certainly not alone! We all feel sorry for ourselves from one time to another. It's almost comforting in a way, isn't it? Secretly that is, like if we don't feel sorry for ourselves, who will? Someone's got to do it, might as well be us? Who can feel sorrier for us, than us? Of course we feel sorry for ourselves! What kind of question is that? Wouldn't we all want to eat a two pound box of chocolates and not gain an ounce? It could happen you know... But not to one of us! The reason I brought this up is because by our very nature, this truly is the way we feel. We feel like we are giving up some thing other people don't have to give up. And it's not just a little something, it's a big something, because the world revolves around it and we are tired of it!

We are tired of not being able to be like everyone else! Am I right? OK! If we are going to feel sorry for ourselves, let's just do it for five minutes a day and let's make sure that no one sees us do it, because after all, it's non-productive. It doesn't look good and it doesn't encourage a positive attitude! Indeed! We should stop and count our blessings daily. My guess is that if we take the time to count the blessings we do have, we will find that they far out weigh the ones we don't have!

I hope that we are starting to become acquainted, because I am about to take you to my "private pantry" where I have learned over the years to "create and compensate". It has a rather nice ring to it doesn't it?

I had a revelation which was... That if any of these recipes could help just one person, make one little change to enhance their life in any way, I would feel that this book has been a success. I wish I would have had some one out there who would have shared this with me years ago. Many of the carb-junkie friends I have shared these recipes with have urged me to share them with everyone. Of course, sharing is what life is all about.

The object of this book is not to tell you to cut out all of the carbohydrates in your life. I can not tell you to do that. What this book hopes to accomplish, is to offer you rich, decadent, no-carb, or low-carb alternatives to that plate of hash browns, bag of chips, or box of chocolates. I hope to offer you something wonderful enough to get you to trade in those high empty carbs for, and be happy you did. I hope to offer you something you can live with, one step at a time.

As you will see, this book is not just about eating and looking better, it's about feeling better as well. It's about celebrating life. Living and loving better. Life is a celebration! I have really stressed this point because I feel that we really don't celebrate life as we should. We deserve it! So come along with me and LET'S CELEBRATE!

Because of the fact that I am not promoting a diet plan for obvious reasons, but rather a no-carb, low-carb alternative to supplement your meal plan, I am not going to give you accurate carb counts on each specific recipe in this book. I will tell you that all the recipes I am sharing with you are either no-carb or low-carb which usually means traces. In any case, all of them are good substitutes for high-carb empty foods. If you are wondering how many carbs you should be eating a day, as always, check with your regular physician. I know a lot of people who like to eat around 20 carbs a day and I know a lot of people who eat higher than that. On the other hand, I know of some people who do not eat any at all. I personally do not like to cut them all out. As you get to know the carb count in foods, you will at some point get to know which foods are high and which are low. Aren't we tired of counting anyway? Life is too short.

Look at it this way. Any empty high-carb food that you replace with a low-carb nutritious food is already a good change. The more you make those good changes, the better and easier it gets. Don't deprive yourself. Do it at your own pace, and remember, the more you keep at it, the better the results. Do it so that you can live with it. Build for success!

Let me ask you this... does it all sound too good to be true? I have heard this a few times before. If you are like me you have tried everything, and I mean everything. The reason we have spent so much time spinning our wheels and wasting our precious time (and it's the kind of time that leaves us deflated and depressed), is because there are just no clear cut answers as to who should be doing what! Every "body" is different and it's not the doctor's that are telling us that. You know that you have spent a month trying your girlfriend's diet. The same one she is on at the same time she is on it. It works for her, but not for you. The only thing you have lost in thirty days... is thirty days!

My "diet doctor" didn't tell me this, I had to figure it out on my own. Maybe this will save you a little work and aggravation on your part. I finally joined a group in my area. You know, the large one that let's you count your points and eat whatever you want. I like this group because they seem to have a pretty high success rate. I happen to know some of those successful people. However, there is a snag here. I happen to know some unsuccessful people as well. If you are one of those people who have tried this program and it didn't work for you, and you have read with me so far and decided you are a carb-junkie, I can probably tell you why it didn't work (if you really did stick to it), and how you may be able to make it work, with a simple adjustment in your line of thinking.

Here is what happened to me. I joined the group with absolute excitement. After all, if the Duchess could do it, so could I! The first couple of weeks were very good because I tried to get the most food possible out of my points! Who wouldn't? I tried to stay with just lean meat and a vegetable here and there. It worked! However, after the novelty wore off, and it usually does, I noticed that I started to switch my points over to the high-carb stuff, because we carb-junkies do that naturally. Before you know it, I was using my total daily points on high carb, empty calorie food and what do you think happened? I was eating within my points. I just wasn't losing any weight. In fact, I recall gaining a pound or two here and there. Now, it didn't take a "Rocket Scientist" to figure out that there was something going wrong here, and this is where a lot of people de-rail. This is the point of absolute frustration! This is exactly where most of us quit! It worked for the person next to you, but it's not working for you! You are doing everything they tell you to do and it still isn't working for you! Why? What's wrong with me you say? Why isn't this working for ME? It's becoming so frustrating that now you don't even really want to congratulate the gal who is getting her 25 pound weight loss pin, and now...

Good-bye group! And of course on the way home, you will stop and pick up that burrito you have been craving! Why try? It doesn't work anyway!

Hello there! I re-started spending my points back on the low-carb food, as I had done in the beginning and VIOLA! I was back on track before you know it. This is GOOD news for you my friend, because what this may reveal to you is simple. If you are a carb-junkie and you have tried everything, and all the rest of the stuff here fits you, you may want to try keeping your carbs as low as possible or you just might not be able to lose the weight. Simple enough? Does this make any sense to you? I don't think there are too many other options. I think we are at the end of the road and it only turns right... Right towards some delicious low-carb meals, snacks and desserts. So, follow me!

LET'S START OUT IN THE COTTAGE HOUSE PANTRY

There are a host of treasures waiting to be had here. These are condiments you will want to explore on a wide variety of foods. Flavor is what we are now going to be looking for and if you are bored with the ordinary and would like something wonderful to add to your foods to get that big flavor, try these.

Let's start with some simple yet elegant "Mustards". If you don't care for mustards, don't run away just yet! There are several twists that you can do, that may very well give you a fresh new look at them. Mustards just aren't mustards any more!

Mustards can be used for gift giving. Simply pack them into a lined wicker basket along with a little loaf of bread and a roll of salami, maybe a bottle of wine and you have a perfectly unique and inexpensive gift. They make an even better hostess gift if someone invites you to dinner with a friend. Put them in designer jars, and away you go!

Have you ever thought of using them in a sauce that is rather bland? What an exotic pick-up! If you do not care for mustards because you feel that they are too spicy for you, try cutting them with a little cream or wine and you have a beautiful sauce for your meat, fish, seafood or poultry. You will find that you can add them to just about anything and this is where the fun begins!

MUSTARDS

A little mustard, a lot of flavor! I do not believe that there is a mustard that you can not alter to suit your taste and actually enjoy! You just have to experiment a little. Maybe you would like to add mustard concoctions to your vegetables to heighten their flavor. You really should not pass on these opportunities!

Have you ever thought of using mustards with your cheese platters? Add them to your cheese sauces or spread on crackers. You'll look like you are really in vogue because everything seems to be designer today!

And best of all, these mustards are everything to the hot dog or hamburger lover! You know what they can do for a ham sandwich! To tell you the truth, I never really cared much for mustard until I turned my self into a mustard lover just by coming up with mustards that were pleasing to me. Now I love them.

Cranberry Mustard

    1 cup Dijon style mustard
    1 Tbsp. whole cranberry sauce
    1 pinch cinnamon
    1 pinch coarse salt
    1 pinch allspice

Blend all ingredients well. Spoon into container or designer jar. Cover tightly with lid and refrigerate.

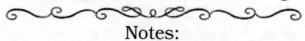

Notes:

Pickle Relish Mustard

1 cup Dijon style or regular mustard
1 Tbsp. pickle relish
¼ tsp. minced garlic

Blend all ingredients and put into container or designer jar. Cover tightly with lid. Refrigerate.

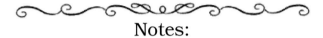

Notes:

Mustard with Horseradish

    1 cup Dijon style mustard
    1 Tbsp. ground horseradish
    1 tsp. minced garlic
    1 pinch allspice
    1 pinch sugar

Mix all ingredients well. Spoon into container or designer jar and cover tightly with lid. Refrigerate.

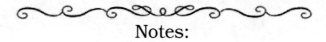

Notes:

Brown Sugar Mustard

    1 cup Dijon style mustard
    2 tsp. brown sugar
    1 pinch allspice
    1 pinch ginger
    1 pinch cinnamon
    1 pinch salt

Mix all ingredients well. Spoon into a container or designer jar. Cover tightly with lid and refrigerate.

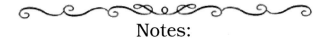

Notes:

Mustard with Peppercorns

1 cup Dijon style mustard
1 Tbsp. crushed peppercorns
pinch of allspice
pinch of cinnamon
¼ tsp. dried tarragon
pinch of coarse salt

Blend all ingredients well. Spoon into container or designer jar. Cover tightly with lid and refrigerate.

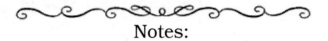

Notes:

Ginger Honey Mustard

1 cup Dijon style mustard
1 Tbsp. honey, any flavor
1 pinch cinnamon
1 pinch ginger
1 pinch salt

Mix well and put into container or designer jar. Cover tightly with lid and refrigerate.

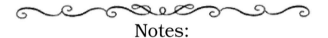

Notes:

Gardner Bob's Pesto Sauce

2 cups fresh basil
½ cup Pine nuts
4 tsp. minced garlic
½ cup Parmesan cheese
½ stick melted butter

Process all ingredients in food processor. Put in container or designer jar. Cover tightly with lid and refrigerate. Makes 1 cup.

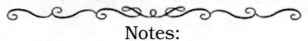

Notes:

Use on meats, add to pasta salads, regular salads, spread on cheese. Add some heavy cream to a couple tablespoons pesto, cook down a little to thicken and it makes a wonderful sauce for vegetables or meats.

Take a piece of deli meat, spread with cream cheese, then spread with pesto. Roll up into a log, slice into pieces and serve. This makes a great appetizer. All pesto and mustards can be put in designer jars with lids. Tie with ribbon or raffine. Add designer label or make your own.

Now you have a great gift!

HERBAL OILS

Let's take a look at infused oils. If you have never tried them before, I urge you to try them. Lot's of big flavor, yum! You can buy them already made or you can make them yourself. Use them for sauté. Add them anywhere oil is called for in a recipe. Use them on vegetables or drizzle on meats before baking in the oven. Use them on salads, the sky is the limit. They will go anywhere your imagination takes you!

Also, remember that the longer infused oils sit around, the more flavorful they will become. These oils also make great gifts if you put them in tall designer bottles, tie with a ribbon or raffine and add a personalized label.

Here are some recipes you might have fun trying. Simple yet elegant!

If you prefer to buy them in the store and I highly suggest that you do try them, they come in flavors that were once unimaginable! The variety is limitless and you can have a ball with them. There are Asian oils, Italian oils, Mexican and Caribbean oils just to name a few! These oils can turn eating vegetables into an experience in and of itself! Remember! Optimum flavor is where it's at!

Dill Oil

1 cup of good olive oil (use only olive oil)
1 Tbsp. dill weed
¼ tsp. salt

Mix well... put in container, store in cool dark place or refrigerate.

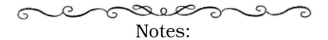

Notes:

Basil Oil

1 cup of good olive oil, (use only olive oil)
1 Tbsp. sweet basil
¼ tsp. salt

Mix well... put in container, store in cool dark place or refrigerate.

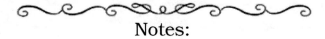

Notes:

Tarragon Oil

1 cup of good olive oil (use only olive oil)
1 tsp. dried tarragon
¼ tsp. salt

Mix well... put in container. Store in a cool dark place or refrigerate.

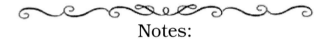

Notes:

Dill Oil

       olive oil, no substitute
       1 tall designer bottle
       fresh dill stocks with heads
       ¼ tsp. salt

Push 3-4 stocks of dill down into the designer bottle at different heights. Add salt... fill with olive oil. Cap and add ribbon or raffine around the neck of the bottle. Add a designer label and store in a cool dark place or refrigerate.

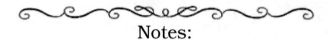

Notes:

Basil Oil

olive oil, no substitute
1 tall designer bottle
fresh basil stocks and leaves
¼ tsp. salt

Push desired amount of fresh basil down into the bottle. Add salt. Fill with olive oil. Cap and put some ribbon or raffine around the neck of the bottle. Add designer label and store in a cool dark place or refrigerate.

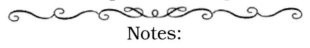

Notes:

Tarragon Oil

olive oil, no substitute
fresh tarragon stocks
1 tall designer bottle
¼ tsp. salt

Push desired amount of tarragon stocks down into the bottle at different levels. Add salt and olive oil. Cap and tie the neck with some ribbon or raffine. Add designer label and store in cool dark place or refrigerate.

Notes:

COTTAGE HOUSE DAIRY

Emile's dairy store herbed butters...

These are an absolute must for your kitchen! Keeping in mind that butter has no carbs, you must add these to your vegetables, sauces, fish, chicken, beef, pork and seafood. Anything and everything! The flavor these butters will add to your dish, you simply can't do without. This is what creating flavor is all about. They add depth, richness and style to just about anything you can eat.

You can also use these butters as fabulous little gift ideas... Hostess gifts, Birthday gifts, Christmas gifts, gifts as a Thank You, or better yet, gifts for no reason. All you have to do is mix them well, put them into a decorative little cheese crock, designer jar or roll them in wax paper or clear wrap. Add a designer label and away you go! This is so much fun!

Want a great tip?... If you are having a dinner party, any one of these flavored butters can be pressed into a large mold, chilled and used as a table decoration. Simply flavor a couple of pounds of butter, press into a large candy or Jello mold and chill. Remove from mold, plate it up, add a garnish and it makes a stunning table decoration that you can eat.

Dill Butter

1 cup butter, softened but not melted
1 tsp. dill weed
½ tsp. minced garlic
2 Tbsp. roasted Pine nuts, optional

Mix well, shape into roll, and wrap or put into crock or lidded container. Decorate with ribbon or raffine if desired. Add designer label.

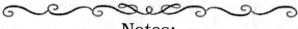

Notes:
TIP: For something fun... spread softened flavored butters into candy molds of any shape you desire. Freeze and when ready to serve... pop out of molds for individual servings or place on serving platter. Makes a wonderful table presentation.

Garlic Butter

1 cup butter, softened but not melted
1 tsp. minced garlic
½ package dry Italian dressing mix
½ tsp. parsley flakes

Mix well, shape into log and wrap or put into lidded container.   Decorate with ribbons or designer label. Refrigerate.

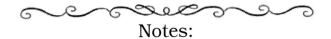

Notes:

Basil Butter

      1 cup butter, softened but not melted
      1 tsp. dried sweet basil leaves
      1 tsp. minced garlic
      2 Tbsp. roasted Pine nuts... optional

Mix well, shape into roll, and wrap or put into crock or lidded container. Decorate with ribbon or raffine if desired. Add designer label.

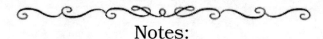

Notes:

TIP: When you sauté mushrooms... If you do not want all the juice to escape the mushrooms, (so that they don't shrivel up to nothing) ... get your sauté pan and oil almost to the point of smoking (high heat) and throw them in at that point. Sauté quickly... Only a couple of minutes. Always watch your heat levels because at the point of smoking, a fire can erupt very quickly. Not failing to mention, alcohol will flame at this point very easily. Remove pan from flame before adding any alcohol, and NEVER add alcohol straight from the bottle to the pan!

Orange Citrus Butter

1 cup butter, softened but not melted
2 tsp. orange zest
2 tsp. lemon zest
2 Tbsp. orange juice or 1 tsp. Grand Marnier

Mix well, shape into roll, and wrap or put into crock or lidded container. Decorate with ribbon or raffine if desired. Add designer label.

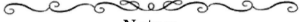

Notes:
Great on vegetables, seafood, and chicken.

Mo Jo Butter

1 cup butter, softened not melted
2 tsp. lime zest
1 Tbsp. honey
1 tsp crushed red pepper flakes
2 Tbsp. lime juice
¼ tsp. cayenne pepper

Mix well, shape into roll, and wrap or put into crock or lidded container. Decorate with ribbon or raffine if desired. Add designer label.

Notes:
Great for corn on the cob...

Pecan or Walnut Butter

1 cup butter, softened but not melted
½ cup chopped pecans or walnuts
2 Tbsp. brown sugar

Mix well, shape into roll, and wrap or put into crock or lidded container. Decorate with ribbon or raffine if desired. Add designer label.

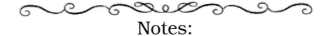

Notes:

Honey Butter

1 cup butter, softened but not melted
1 Tbsp. honey

Mix well, shape into roll, and wrap or put into crock or lidded container. Decorate with ribbon or raffine if desired. Add designer label.

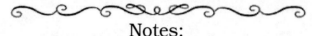

Notes:

TIP: Whenever cooking... Get all of your ingredients measured, chopped, diced and ready to go before you start your cooking project. You won't believe how much easier it makes the whole process. Keep a garbage container (bowl) right on the counter for all of the little odds and ends. This makes throwing the trash on the counter away a lot easier!

Horseradish Butter

1 stick of butter, room temperature
3 Tbsp. brown mustard
1 Tbsp. horseradish

Place in bowl, beat until creamy. Serve room temperature. Mix well, shape into roll, and wrap or put into crock or lidded container. Decorate with ribbon or raffine if desired. Add designer label.

Notes:
Melt on top of vegetables or meat. Refrigerate leftovers.

Chili Butter

1 stick butter, room temperature
2 Tbsp. hot sauce
1 tsp. chili powder
½ tsp. minced garlic

Mix well, shape into roll, and wrap or put into crock or lidded container. Decorate with ribbon or raffine if desired. Add designer label.

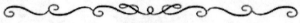

Notes:
Goes especially well with corn on the cob.

Herbed Butter

1 stick butter, room temperature
2 Tbsp. chopped chives
1 Tbsp. Worcestershire sauce
1 tsp. dried sweet basil
1 tsp. dried dill
½ tsp. coarse salt

Mix well, shape into roll, and wrap or put into crock or lidded container. Decorate with ribbon or raffine if desired. Add designer label.

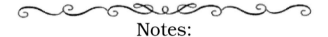

Notes:

In France, everyone knows the beauty of Crème Fraiche. This is an ultra-rich version of sour cream. Much thicker, much richer, much smoother and less tangy than sour cream. Use it plain or add any herb you desire to it and let the flavors meld together before using. Add it to meat sauces, gravies and stews to add a richer flavor. Melt over vegetables. Use your imagination. It works especially well with chicken, fish and pork.

Here is all you do to be able to have this rich cream in your own home, because sometimes it is not too easy to find in the market. Recipe follows.

Ettie Bickford's Crème Fraiche

To one cup of heavy cream... you add 3 tablespoons of buttermilk. Put into glass jar with lid. Mix well. Let sit at room temperature for 24 hours. Then stir and refrigerate. This is so good!

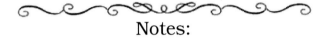

Notes:

Here are some variations that you can do with your Crème. This is so much fun. To your Crème Fraiche you can add a tablespoon of lime juice and chopped cilantro and use for tacos or fish. Use ANY herb you love and mix well. Add a combination and see what happens. Add a tablespoon of orange juice, some orange zest and a little honey and you have a topping for fruit. Use lemon the same way. Place a couple of tablespoons of sugar-free butterscotch or caramel ice cream topping into it and you have a decadent fruit dip. Add a package of dry Italian dressing mix and you have a wonderful dip for vegetables, the list goes on and on.

TIP: Once you get the hang of this, you will always be able to have it on hand. It's much less expensive than buying it in the store. It is much fresher and there are many variations. Add cheese and bacon... instant Egg Wrap topping!

GETTING TO KNOW YOUR CHEESES

Let's start by saying that if cheese is going to be another staple in our new life style, let's not get bored with this either. I think you are going to have to learn something about cheeses. Really experiment with them. Try things that you never would have tried before. If you know all about cheeses great! If not, read on.

Here is what I would call a good "starter kit" and you can take it from there. I believe that you can get a lot of mileage out of the flavor of a good cheese. I am sorry, but I know people who have never known that there was a cheese life beyond American, cheddar and mozzarella. Maybe they have ventured into the provolone or the Monterey Jack, but, very limited. If you like cheese... do you have any idea what you are missing? Even if you don't like cheese you might be missing something. I hope you are not judging the taste of cheese on the American or low fat American cheese in the dairy section of the grocery store! One of our favorites is Jarlsberg, it's incredible. It is the best on a meat platter and it does wonders for a fruit platter as well.

A heavenly host of cheeses are available at your local market these days. We have it much better now than we did years ago because cheeses from all over the world are available to us now. The beauty of a good cheese shop, and I would recommend a trip to a good cheese shop just because it is fun, is that the wonderful people at the cheese shops will let you taste the cheese before you buy it! Ergo! It takes the guess work out of what to buy. That is the best way to do it. If you guess at the store, you might wind up with a moldy chunk of cheese and a bad attitude! You might say, "See, I tried it and I don't like it." We do not want that!

Here is a simple guide to some of the most popular cheeses.

From France... "Brie" is a buttery soft cheese with a white edible rind. It's cream colored interior is very soft, even slightly runny at the peak of ripeness. Brie can also be found flavored with herbs, peppercorns or garlic. Brie is excellent served warm with fresh fruits, vegetables or meat for dipping.

"Port Salute"... is a smooth soft cheese that has a creamy yellow interior. It's flavor can range from mild to robust. In any flavor, it is a good choice for an appetizer tray.

"Roquefort" Frances "Blue Cheese", is an ivory white cheese with blue or grey veins running throughout. It has a firm crumbly texture and a full hearty flavor. Crumble on salads or serve with fruits and meats.

From Denmark... "Havarti"... is a semi-soft pale yellow cheese. It's creamy texture is filled with tiny little holes. Havarti has a mild flavor which may be flavored with dill or caraway. Tilsit is an aged havarti with a more intense flavor and a firmer texture. Both are delicious table cheeses.

"Danish Blue"... is a creamy, crumbly, blue veined cheese. Good in salads, dips, dressings and sauces. Delicious served with fruits such as pears or apples.

From Greece... "Feta"... is a salty crumbly white cheese that is very dry. It's popularity has soared and given rise to flavored feta cheeses such as sun-dried tomato, peppercorn and pesto. Good in salads or on bruchetta.

"Mizithra"... is a firm dry cheese made from goat, sheep or cows milk. Salty and distinctly tangy, this white cheese is delicious grated and served with Olive oil as a dip.

From Italy... "Parmigano Reggiano"... is one of Italy's oldest cheeses and probably one of the most beloved in any Italian cuisine. This hard cheese with a granular texture has a robust flavor. Pale in color, Parmigano Reggiano can be used as a grating cheese or table cheese. (This is what I use in any recipe that calls for Parmesan cheese... it's the best!).

"Asiago"... like many cheeses has many personalities. Young asiago cheese can be used as a table cheese or used for melting and is wonderful in cream sauces. Aged Asiago should be used as a grating cheese. Asiago has a rich nutty flavor that resembles a cross between sharp cheddar and Parmesan.

"Fresh Mozzarella"... is packaged in water or whey unlike regular mozzarella, which is semi-soft and elastic in texture. Fresh mozzarella has a softer texture and a sweet delicate flavor. Serve sliced with fresh tomatoes, freshly chopped basil and a drizzle of olive oil.

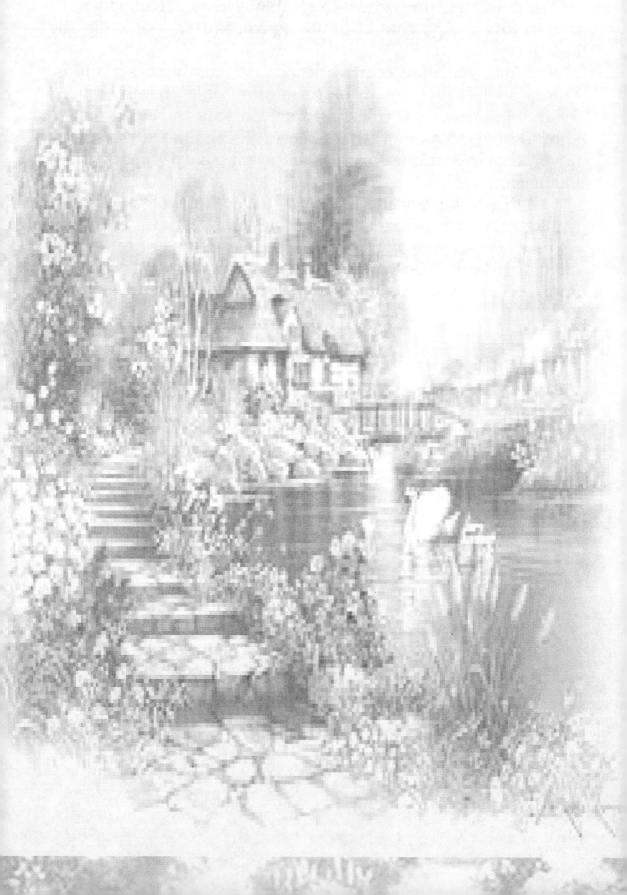

LESSONS FROM THE COTTAGE HOUSE

Let's take a break from the recipes for a moment and talk about our daily lives. At the Cottage House we have a random gift giving day once a month. At the beginning of the month we put little squares of paper in a bowl. Each paper has a day of the month written on it, so that all the days in the month are covered. Each of us then picks a square with a day on it and that is our day to do something special for someone. Someone we may not know very well. Someone who may be going through a hard time, it doesn't matter. We hand make something or buy some little trinket and give it with heart-felt enthusiasm.

This is fun to do. It does not even have to be for a particular reason. These are just little rays of sunshine. It doesn't take much to do these little gestures, but it surely does make a big impact on someone's day. Not only that, I believe that it makes most of us feel really good to do something nice for someone else. Try it for yourself and see.

If you want to make a little gift for someone else or just for yourself, try this. It's absolutely wonderful and it will make the gift receiver feel really special!

Into a quart-sized food storage bag, add two cups of cornstarch and several drops of scented essential oil. Some suggestions would be lavender, rose, peppermint, sage, honeysuckle, lilac, or foxglove. Use your imagination. Give it a good shake. Close bag with a pretty ribbon and label it with a designer label. Place name of the fragrance on the label. Put it in a designer box if desired. Personalize it by adding a name. Use this after a bath or shower. You can also use it to simply refresh yourself on a hot summer day. What an inexpensive and wonderful gift. Add a little puff pad to dust the body with and away you go!

HERE ARE A FEW TIPS:

Did you know...? That if you squeeze the juice of a lemon onto a musty smelling dish cloth, the odor vanishes immediately? Use the juice of a lemon to sanitize your counter tops and butcher blocks. It's said to kills germs as well as any cleanser can, but it's so safe you can eat it. Simply rub half a lemon all over the counter tops and wipe clean. After all, the chemicals that you get on your skin go into your blood.

You will shed fewer tears while cutting onions, if you cut the root end of the onion off first. And of course, keep your onions cold.

I know people who do not particularly like the idea of eating chunks of onion in their burgers or meat loaf. To get the flavor of onion with out the chunks, grate the onion with a grater. Not only will you not get the chunks, you will add moisture to your meat.

Always stand your asparagus upright in a container of water in your refrigerator. It will add twice as much life as storing them in a food storage bag.

When mixing something that requires multiple eggs, crack them into a separate bowl before adding them to the mix. If you happen to get a bad egg, you won't ruin the whole recipe.

Try this once... As a stress reliever, have someone rub Peppermint Essential Oil (therapeutic grade) onto the back of your neck, shoulder blades and perhaps the tops of your shoulders as well. Take a few deep breaths and see what happens! Quality Essential Oils are KEY here. Once you can feel the coolness, rotate your arms gently and then let them drop to your sides as loosely as possible. The effect is awesome. Who needs an aspirin anyway!

Always remember... There are no real victims in life, only students. We are always learning!

MORE FROM THE COTTAGE HOUSE

We need to talk about cream sauces. For those of you who do not particularly care for those yummy cream sauces on your meats, vegetables, eggs, seafood or poultry, you might want to read this section anyway. You just never know when you might want to expand your horizons.

Isn't an adventurous life all about trying new things? Or like mom always told me, at least give it a chance before you tell me that you don't like it! Maybe I should thank Mom for my sense of adventure.

Slathering on those wonderful sauces, to me, is yet another way of enhancing flavors. And as I have said again and again, that is what most of us need to succeed! Remember, it's all about what we are willing to give up the carb for, and it better be tasty!

There are many types of sauces to choose from and you certainly don't always have to use them. To me, it just makes me feel like I'm not giving up so much on the other end!

Although these sauces are rich and tasty, you can get by with eating them because they have very few carbs, or none at all! Of course, they do have calories so use your best judgment. With sauces, you can get by with using smaller amounts, so what's the problem? I really urge you to try them. It adds a whole new dimension to your entrée.

Are we ready to let loose a little? Get a little adventureous? Get the most out of our meal?

Good, because it's show time!!! We are going to be working with three different sauces which have many variations. All of these are easy to make and fun to work with.

In fact, there are so many variations in what you can do with these sauces, that once you get the hang of it, your friends and family will be calling you the "sauce queen" or the "sauce king"! and you will derive great satisfaction in sharing your recipes with them.

However, before we get into the sauces, we simply must discuss the sauces' counter-parts, the herbs and spices. You are going to have to know a little something about these guys. If you do already, that's great. If you don't, read on!

You are going to have to get a little friendly with the herb and spice sections at your favorite market. In fact, you can get a little friendly with the butcher as well, but that comes in later on. Don't get nervous. It's not as bad as it sounds! I can give you a little help here, but pretty soon, you won't even need me. Experimentation is really the name of the game here. Who knows, you might like this herbing and spicing so much that it will make you forget that you ever wanted to eat big carbs in the first place. We can all crave personal gratification even more than we crave food, so why not get our gratification from impressing all of our friends and family with our ingeniously tasty recipes instead of a bag of chips? It's much more productive this way and it feels a whole lot better!

I always recommend that you use fresh herbs and spices whenever possible. You just get the optimum flavor this way. However, if this is not an option, don't get nervous. The bottled and bagged will work too. The big problem with bottled is that once opened, it starts to lose it's potency. One step in the right direction would be to simply buy your bottled spices in the smallest containers possible. Have you ever pulled out a can of poultry seasoning that you know for absolute sure has been in your cupboard since you got married, oh, say... 20 years ago? You know who you are and you're not alone. What color was that supposed to be? Does it look so bad now that you can't tell if it is actually spice or dust? You certainly could never tell by the smell, because there isn't any left!

And what's up with the gallon of cilantro you bought at the store a while ago because it was on sale? Yes, this is for you Jackie! My friend Jackie, who I have heard on more than a couple of occasions say that she was not particularly fond of this vivacious herb, went and bought a quantum jar because her recipe called for it and it was on sale. This stuff will spawn new life forms before she ever uses it again... and it's taking up huge space on the top shelf of her cabinet! This is NOT a good thing!

To start out simply, this is what I could suggest as a "starter kit" in the herb department. If you are going to use the bottled, start out with basil, thyme, rosemary, tarragon, dill, sage and marjoram. This is a simple starter kit. There are dozens of other herbs, but for now, keep it simple and when you get the hang of it go exploring. Maybe buy a good book on herbs. I also chose these herbs because in the fresh, they are readily available in the local markets. During the growing season the open markets are the most wonderful places to buy your fresh herbs. You can buy them growing in containers. Take them home and continue to let them grow in your window or on your patio and have them fresh whenever needed.

Here is what I would suggest as a simple "starter kit" of spices to have on hand. Start out with kosher or coarse salt, peppercorns for the pepper mill, paprika, curry powder, cayenne pepper and maybe a couple of your favorite season salt blends. If you really want to shake things up a little, try checking out all the different peppercorn blends that they have in the stores now. I personally really like the Caribbean spice blends. These could be a whole separate book. You see, this stuff just keeps getting better all the time. While I'm on the subject, get your self a good pepper mill and grind your own peppercorns. Throw out the pre-ground pepper! You'll be glad you did! The difference in flavor is astounding!

Always have the trio on hand. What trio? Carrots, celery and onions. But don't forget the garlic! Garlic... garlic... garlic! You can never have enough garlic. This is standard fare for a great stock. Veal, pork, chicken or beef. I try to make my own stock from scratch, but if you are going to buy it in the store, try to get it in a can. None of that granular stuff please! If you really want to go all out, you can buy some saffron, but saffron is expensive. Expensive but worth it. Turmeric may be used as a substitute for the color of saffron but you won't get the flavor.

As far as wines and vinegars go, I would say if you like the taste of it use it. Rule of thumb, if you wouldn't drink it, you probably shouldn't cook with it. Whatever you do, please try not to buy the cooking wines in the grocery store. You know, the ones next to the vinegars? They don't even qualify! Here are some simple suggestions to start out with. I think a good Marsala, Madeira, Dry or Cream Sherry or a Cabernet Sauvignon and once again, when you get the hang of it, use whatever you like! The sky is the limit! A couple of the vinegars would be a champagne vinegar, a rice wine vinegar, a good balsamic vinegar and then explore for yourself. Above all, enjoy yourself and have fun. Don't worry about mistakes. Everybody makes them. It's part of learning! Some of the greatest creations have come from mistakes. They have tons of flavored oils and vinegars in the stores. Why not have some fun with them?

ON TO THE SAUCES

The first sauce... A simple "cream sauce". This is a sauce that you will be making from the pan drippings of a meat dish that you have just completely prepared and removed from the oven, stove or broiler. First, you will want to remove your meat from the pan, leaving all of the drippings and brown bits. If you have excess grease in the pan, you may want to pour a little of it off and discard it. Next you will want to de-glaze the pan by setting it on the burner with a medium low flame and adding about ¼ - ½ cup liquid. This liquid could be wine, stock, or a vinegar such as champagne vinegar, what ever flavor you think would compliment your dish. Bring this to a simmer and scrape all the particles from the bottom of the pan. At this point, you may want to season with salt or pepper or some other spice (never add fresh herbs until the very end). Now you can go ahead and add scallions, garlic, or even mushrooms if you desire. Let them cook down a little. Now you are ready to add your cream. I usually add roughly 1½ cups of heavy cream and simmer until the sauce is reduced and thickened to a point I am satisfied with. If you are using a vinegar in the sauce add it to taste, because they have a stronger flavor than beef stock or wine. You might want to check your sauce now to see if you have to add any additional spices and if you don't, you are good to go! Drizzle it on your dish. It should be very tasty. If it isn't, you will need to work on it a little longer. Play around and have some fun. Be creative!

TIP: Some other things you might like to try adding to your sauce would be diced roma tomatoes, diced yellow, orange or red bell pepper for color, or bacon bits. I have even used baby shrimp and dill if I am going to be using my sauce for fish or seafood along with the diced roma tomatoes. I've also used a sauce with shrimp in it to smother my steak!

TIP: I always like to garnish my plates with a fresh herb or parsley. You can sprinkle on minced parsley or even sweet Paprika for a little color. Don't stop there! In no time, you will be surprised at what you can garnish a plate with. It should definitely be a work of art... you need to appeal to the visual as well.

TIP: Always make your plate look attractive for a nice presentation.

TIP: You can use your sauce under your meat, or on top of your meat. You can even dabble some sauce around the edge of the plate before you garnish. It looks so nice! Make some garnishes out of vegetables and add them to your plate. There are inexpensive books in the stores that show you how to do this. It's great fun and it doesn't take a "rocket scientist" either! I always find that the more attractive the plate looks, the better the food tastes to me, and the more satisfied I feel. Eating should be a visual as well as a tasty experience. To me it's like opening the prettiest wrapped Birthday gift. You just go for it because you can't help yourself... you can't resist! The package is exciting!

Did you know...? That the best gift you can give someone is to make them feel really important and it doesn't cost you a cent? I just love it when I go into a restaurant and one of the owner's or manager's call me by my name. You know that you are just "one of the customers" but it still makes you feel important.

The next thing we are going to talk about is a "roux".
A "roux" is a sauce thickener. These are used in everything
from sauces and soups to stews, gumbos, gravies and more.
Something to consider about a roux is that it is made with
flour, and flour contains some carbs. I personally feel that
the carbs are low enough by the time everything is
distributed that I do not worry about it. What you need to
do to make a roux, is in a medium skillet, add equal parts
of flour and vegetable oil. I even use butter. Next you will
want to make a paste by mixing it thoroughly over low heat.
Now you will be ready to add your liquid. Before we go on
to making the sauce by adding the liquid, let me finish
explaining about the "roux", because there is more to learn
here. If you only want to make one cup of sauce made with
"roux", you use one tablespoon of flour mixed with one
tablespoon vegetable oil brought together in a paste in a
skillet and now you are ready to add liquid. However, you
can also make a roux in quantity, taste and color. This is a
good idea to do ahead of time so that you always have it on
hand. You can change the taste and color of a roux by the
length of time you simmer it. This allows your roux to go
from very light tasting and light colored to nutty flavored
and dark colored. How you want to develop your roux
depends on what you will be using it for. Lighter color and
flavor used in light sauces and of course darker roux used
in heavier soups, stews, gumbos and gravies where you
would like a deeper color and depth of flavor. Now, let's go
on to talk about the quantity. A nifty little trick I learned
that has come in really handy is to make a big batch of
roux. Put it in ice cube trays, freeze it, and once frozen into
cubes, remove them and place in freezer container. One of
those cubes will make one cup of sauce. How convenient
and you will always have them on hand! Drop it in and give
it a stir. It just doesn't get any easier or faster than that! I
suppose you are thinking by now, she didn't tell me how to
get that dark color in the roux?

Well, here we go! There are a couple of ways to do this. The first way is to add flour and oil, (and I usually use one cup of flour to one cup oil) to a skillet to make a paste, making sure it is blended well. Keep the heat low and spread mixture out over the bottom of the pan. Simmer very slowly until color starts to get darker. Keep simmering until you get the color you want. Do not go too dark on the color because if you go too far, it will burn and become bitter. The color should be anywhere from a light brown to a mahogany with a nice nutty fragrance. If you would like the roux a light color, you do not have to simmer it at all, just get it blended and refrigerate or freeze. Another way to do this would be to put two cups of flour into a pie plate and the next time you are baking a roast, just put it in the oven on the other rack and bake until the flour turns the color you desire making sure not to burn it. You can bake it on it's own but why waste the gas? Once you get the color you desire you can then add it to two cups of vegetable oil to make a paste and refrigerate or freeze.

Now, what do I do with this roux? There are many things to do with it, but as we are concentrating on sauces, we are going to do sauces. I am going to give you a few examples of what you can do starting out with the light roux.

To one cube of light roux, you can add one cup of milk and it will make a white sauce. To that you can add anything you desire, be it cheese, paprika, cayenne, hot sauce, chopped hard boiled eggs, tuna, red, yellow, orange or green diced bell peppers... Whatever floats your boat! Be creative!

To one cube of light roux, you can add one cup of chicken stock and you will have a nice chicken gravy or sauce. Try adding beef stock, veal stock or vegetable stock.

Take a cube of light roux, and add it to a soup or stew to thicken, keeping in mind that one cube will thicken one cup of liquid.

Use your darker roux to make gravies, sauces, stews, soups and gumbos using the same technique. Remember it is up to your taste in seasoning these sauces once thickened. Use them any way you like. Once again, let your imagination run wild!

TIP: You can always use the pan drippings from your meat to start your roux. Simply drop a cube into the pan drippings, blend well and add your cup of liquid what ever it will be or any combination there of. Season and enjoy! You can use wine or champagne vinegar for this sauce as well.

TIP: If you would like to try an awesome cheese sauce, my personal favorite... (which really rocks) on vegetables, scrambled eggs, even fish, here's how you make it.

To 1½ cups of heavy cream, you add ¾ cup any kind of creamy, easy to melt cheese (I use American for this sauce), 1 tsp. dry or regular mustard, and any hot sauce or cayenne pepper to taste. Blend well and simmer until sauce thickens to desired consistency. It will thicken without a thickening agent, but it may take a few minutes. This is so good!

The next sauce we want to talk about is a "natural" sauce. A natural sauce does not have a thickening agent but can be made every bit as tasty. Natural sauces are especially good on fish, seafood, salmon or any meat for that matter. Try them on vegetables as well.

Again, this sauce is made by de-glazing the pan you prepared your meat in with some stock, wine, vinegar, or any combination. Scrape all the browned bits off the bottom of the pan. At this point you can add any herbs, spices, onions, garlic, mushrooms, diced roma tomatoes, whatever you feel comfortable using. Reduce liquid a little. Remove from heat and add a couple of tablespoons of butter to smooth it out and pour over meat, fish, seafood or vegetables and enjoy!

Well, how do you like this so far? Have we been able to help you at all? Do you think you could have a little fun with this? I really urge you to try some of these things because they really do maximize the flavor of your food!

I feel like we are starting to become a little acquainted here, so let's continue on our journey together into... what's next? Dips... rich creamy dips!

Did you know...? The best way I know of to acquire a good friend, is to be a good friend. The way I feel about my friends... Priceless!

Always remember...
Life is like a bank account... no deposit... no return!

ON TO THE DIPS

Dips are another staple we want to talk about. These dips are going to play largely into the scheme of things because we carb-junkies need to be heavily armed when it comes to "snack time", the downfall of most of us. Ergo, it is best to be prepared. Friends, if you are like me, when you have to start thinking about what to eat you run into trouble, and snack time is the worst place to be in trouble.

You may want to make a few of these dips on your appetizer making night so that you will have them on hand all week. Keeping these on hand minimizes the risk of running into trouble because you don't have anything made up ahead of time to eat when the snack attack hits. These are also good to have on hand in case you have guests that drop in. Easy snack! Already made! Less temptation to order that pizza! You would be surprised how many things there are to dip. Just make sure to keep them on hand as well. We will get into that later. Before we get dipping, we need to address some personal issues.

We are creatures of convenience. How many times have we gone to the grocery store, took a look around and bought things that required little or no effort to make, regardless of what our intentions were before we got to the store? We know who we are don't we? How many choices do we have in a convenience store? Until recently, you could hardly find a banana by the check out counter and it's really not that much better now. The problem is, I'll bet that is where we spend a good deal of time gassing up the car. Before work, after work, running the kids around on an empty stomach. We've been running around all day doing errands. No time to eat! By that time we have absolutely no sense of good judgment because our stomachs are screaming for nourishment and by golly, it's going to be a candy bar and that can of soda because it's right there in front of you in the check out line and isn't that just the natural selection of things? Besides, you can eat them in the car and you don't even have to wait until you get home! Instant gratification. That's the beauty!

Are you like me? Do you get tired of the glamour queens who have never been more than 15 pounds over their goal weight telling you how to use a thigh master? I'm just curious! Assuring you that if you just do what they tell you to do, you will look like them in no time? It doesn't make me want to use a thigh master, it makes me want to eat a jelly doughnut just on general principle! But friends, this is what we have to contend with on a daily basis and for most of us, this is not reality. Yet, we keep buying the stuff and loosing more altitude. Why try to build abs and pecks when you can't find them anyway? No one really understands us do they? "Just get a thigh master, you'll be fine!" "Just get out there and do a little walking, it will come right off!" Sounds like that one came straight from Mom right? Wouldn't it make more sense to lose some of it first and then tone it up? Maybe a little exercise along the way would be nice, but let's face it friends, exercise is not that much fun when you don't have any one to do it with. Come to think of it, it's not that much fun when you DO have someone to do it with either! Don't laugh! You know most of us think this way, because if we didn't, we wouldn't be in this boat.

How much time do you really spend on yourself? I suspect that you are like me. Are you so busy doing for everyone else that you don't have time for yourself, and even if you did, you would be to exhausted to use it anyway?

We need to start spending a little more time on ourselves, because the last person we need to let us down is us! People will not dislike us because we spend a little time on ourselves, contrary to popular belief. (ours, of course!). Do we secretly think we are little Florence Nightingales' because we are sure that no one can survive with out us?

(If we only had that much control when it came to our own lives!) TRUST ME! The world will go on without us for a little while every week! In fact, people would probably start liking us a little more because WE would start liking us a little more, and this is a good thing if we are going to start depending on ourselves a little bit. We probably wouldn't be as frustrated if our dream of a few moments for ourselves wasn't shattered by the reality that we really could take them if we wanted to, but we don't! Why do we let ourselves come last? Are we getting something out of this? We must be, but what? Why is it more important for us to go over and spend time letting the neighbor's dog out for them, so that they can go do something nice for themselves? Is there something wrong with this picture? It's only the right thing to do, to be good to other people, but friends, we are fantastic people, so let's be good to ourselves as well. I have had a running joke with myself forever. The saying goes..."If I were as good to my friends as I am to myself, they probably wouldn't stick around very long would they?" Now, reflect on that for just a moment!

I have a neighbor, let's call him Ed. 365 days a year, Ed goes out and jogs from 5-7 p.m. Rain, snow, sleet or hail... 50 below zero or 95 above... Ed is out jogging from 5-7 p.m. Ed is married and has children yet at home. One day Ed's wife asked me if I could drop one of the children off at the local high school. I apologized that I could not do it because I was already running late myself. I asked her if Ed could possibly do it. Do you know what she told me? She said, "I couldn't possibly ask Ed, because Ed is out jogging. That's Ed's time for himself. He needs it because his job is so stressful. No one ever asks Ed to do anything in that window of time because they know how committed he is to his jogging". Well now, to the best of my recollection, no one that I know in the neighborhood has ever been angry at Ed for jogging between 5-7 p.m. In fact, everyone adores Ed. They just happen to know what Ed does every night between 5-7 p.m. Do you see the moral to the story? Ed has not lost a friend yet! You won't either!

You probably think by now that I have forgotten about the "dips", but I haven't! And, I'll bet you are wondering why I have been going on and on about spending time on ourselves, right? Well, because the very essence of success right now, is going to depend on a little time commitment from you! Do not be afraid of a little time commitment. We are going to turn this into an adventure that will be worth the time you invested in it. This little time commitment is going to allow us to do some serious preparation work and some diligent planning, which in turn is going to encourage us to make smart and fun choices on our journey to success. What do I mean by all of this? We are going to plan and make all of our up and coming snacks for the whole week, so that we do not even have to think about what to make or eat when we are tired and using poor judgment. Remember, that's how we get into trouble in the first place, when we have to think on an empty, tired stomach. Problem solved!

I would like to think that we are going to become so creative and so proficient at doing this that we would be able to go into business doing it for other people, but right now we are just concerned about our snacks.

You like to get together with your friends right? Grab a friend and do this together. It wouldn't hurt your friend either and after all, two heads are better than one when it comes to brainstorming ideas, right? Get a group of friends together and have a few laughs. Think about having a snack exchange like some people have cookie exchanges at Christmas time. We are having fun already! How about this... The next time your man has his card game or football party, the snacks will already be done! If loved one needs to lose that little beer belly anyway, we've just killed two birds with one stone! Put him to work making these appetizers with you, call it quality time and he'll be burning calories with you to boot! Pretty soon he will be hooked on them too! Oh! By the way, did you know that beef jerky has no or very little carbs? Pretty soon it will be good bye nacho chips! And "guys", pork rinds in the bag? Not a carb to be found. Get your guy on the fast track too! Keep getting your friends involved in this appetizer making thing.

On the following pages I am going to share with you some of the richest, tastiest snacks and dips I could come up with. Naturally, as time goes on, you and your friends will find and create many of your own recipes. Have a contest. See who can come up with the best recipe. Have a cook-off! Come up with a prize! Try and make it fun. Bring your snacks to "food day" at work. Get your co-workers hooked. Pretty soon they will be bringing them to work and you can have a healthier food day. Plus, you will have the energy to finish off the work day instead of being loaded down with carbs and ready for that afternoon nap at your desk!   Make it fun!   It's all in you your attitude! Remember... it's not important to do what you like, but more so to like what you do, so, let's get doing!

Mad Jack's Vegetable Patch Dip

In a food processor, as finely as possible, chop ½ carrot, ½ green pepper, ½ yellow pepper, ½ red pepper and ¼ onion.

Next, mix:
1 cup Mayo (not Miracle Whip)
1 cup sour cream
1 tsp. dill weed
1 tsp. dried parsley
½ tsp. minced garlic
½ tsp. season salt

Then take ½ cup or more of the processed vegetables and put them onto a paper towel. Blot out any excess water. Finally, fold the vegetables into the Mayo mixture and chill... preferably overnight.

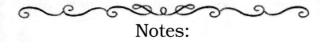

Notes:

Try this unique recipe from a gardener friend of ours...

What do you do with left over veggies? Dip them of course!

Wondering what else to dip? Try slices of turkey, ham, roast beef, chicken, shrimp and even imitation crab or lobster meat. Dip isn't just for veggies anymore!

You can also spoon this delicious dip onto omelets or inside of them. Thin them out a little with cream and drizzle over steamed veggies, fish, chicken or seafood.

Crazy Cucumber Dipping Sauce

½ cup Mayo (not Miracle Whip)
½ cup sour cream
½ cup cucumber, finely diced, and patted dry
1 tsp. finely chopped cilantro
½ tsp finely chopped mint
1 tbsp. lime juice
1 tbsp. orange juice
¼ - ½ tsp minced garlic
salt to taste

Mix ingredients well and refrigerate until ready to use.

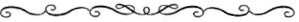

Notes:
This one goes well with MaMa Chula's Jerk Chicken Breasts.

Cottage Vineyard's Sun-Dried Tomato Basil Dip

First, drain one small jar of sun-dried tomatoes. Put them into a paper towel and blot off any extra oil. Next, take ½ jar of olives, slice and pat dry. Dice tomatoes and olives as small as you can get them. Mix them all together with:

> 1 cup Mayo (not Miracle Whip)
> 1 cup sour cream
> 2 tsp. sweet basil
> ½ to 1 tsp. minced garlic
> ¼ tsp. salt

Next... add tomatoes and olives and blend well. Chill.

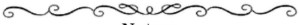

Notes:

Try spreading this on deli slices of ham, roast beef, turkey or Chicken. Roll them up like a wrap, secure with a tooth pick and you have the perfect snack.

TIP: All of these dips can be used any where your imagination can take you. If you wish to thin them out for a sauce, add a little cream and heat. Be creative and see what you can come up with.

Note: Try using a silk flower as a garnish on your plate. Make sure to cut the stem off of it. Pansies are nice. Hibiscus flowers in vibrant colors are very dramatic!

Note: Use very colorful plates and accessories at your lunch or dinner table. You can find them at reduced prices in the thrift stores.

Mrs. Thatcher's Most Excellent Beau Monde Dip

1 cup Mayonnaise (not Miracle Whip)
1 cup sour cream
1 Tbsp. parsley
1 Tbsp. dried onion flakes
1 Tbsp. Beau Monde seasoning
1 tsp. dill weed

Mix well. Chill and serve. Use with vegetables. Add to omelets, dip pork rinds, spread on turkey slices and roll up. Dip cooked chicken tenderloins or nuggets, rolled up pastrami, roast beef or turkey. Refrigerate left-overs.

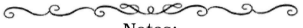

Notes:

What could be easier than this and the flavor only improves the longer it sits during the week!

This is a Cottage House favorite... hands down!

Crazy Carlos' Chile Dip

1 ½ cups Mayo (not Miracle Whip)
½ cup sour cream
2 Tbsp. bottled chili sauce
1 tsp. Splenda
1 tsp. paprika
½ cup chopped black olives
½ to 1 small diced jalapeno, chopped fine
¼ tsp. cayenne pepper

Mix well. Chill.

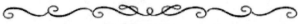

Notes:

Serve with chicken nuggets, chicken wings, and vegetables or add to an omelet for a little zing. Add a couple of tablespoons to eggs before you cook them, or thin out the sauce and pour on top of the omelet when it is done. Garnish with black olives and tomatoes if you wish.
We have thinned this out with a little cream... heated it up a little and served it over scrambled eggs. Yummy! You can even top the scrambled eggs with cheddar cheese and more black olives.

Here is a dip that is just plain fun and tasty. It's a party hit that you just won't find anywhere else.

Did you know...? That submerging a lemon or lime in hot water for 15 minutes or in the microwave for 15 seconds before you use it will yield nearly twice the amount of juice? Rolling them on the counter will also get the juices working as well.

Rufus Taylor's Tongue Tingling Creamy Hot Sauce

1 cup sour cream
1 cup Mayo (not Miracle Whip)
2/3 cup Parmesan cheese, fresh grated
2 Tbsp. bottled hot sauce
½ to 1 jalapeño pepper, diced very small

In a sauce pan, combine ingredients. Cook and stir over low heat until hot and bubbly. Transfer to serving dish and serve with chicken wings, nuggets etc.

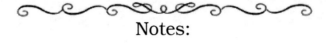

Notes:

If you like it a little on the hot side, and you want a sauce that is served warm. Try this!

Hotsie Totsie Pepper Spread

1 package cream cheese
¼ cup hot pepper jelly
2 Tbsp. chopped green onions

Mix cream cheese with hot pepper jelly (available in most stores). Add chopped green onions. Chill and spread on meats.

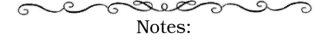

Notes:

Here's a pepper spread you can use on sliced deli meats. Spread on meat, roll up, and secure with a toothpick.

Remember, always check the sugar content in bottled dressings and sauces because some can have carbs, and you may want to account for them. Some of the dressings and sauces may also contain honey.

Are you a roasted vegetable fan? If you've planned ahead like Mrs. Crumby, you will have cut up all sorts of vegetable squares or pieces on your appetizer planning night. When they are cut up ahead of time, all you have to do at the last minute is throw them on a baking dish and away you go. You will need lots of yellow, red, orange and green bell peppers cut up for this one.

Mrs. Crumby's Roasted Vegetables with Tarragon Honey Sauce

Pre-heat the oven to 450 degrees. Spray a jelly roll pan with non-stick spray.

½ lb. fresh green beans
yellow bell pepper wedges
red bell pepper wedges
orange bell pepper wedges
1 lb. sliced or whole mushrooms
2 cups cherry or grape tomatoes
1 cup zucchini sections

Place vegetables in the pan. Drizzle with olive oil, sprinkle with coarse salt and pepper. Add a few pinches of dried tarragon leaves and bake until vegetables are crisp-tender. You can even sprinkle with some freshly grated Parmesan cheese if you wish. Tarragon Honey Sauce recipe follows.

Notes:
Serve warm with dip.

Tarragon Honey Dip

1 cup Mayo (not Miracle Whip)
1 cup sour cream
½ cup Dijon style mustard
1-2 Tbsp. honey
½ tsp. dried tarragon leaves
dash coarse salt

Cover and refrigerate until ready to serve.

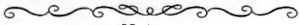

Notes:

Drizzle over veggies right in the pan, or place the dip into a serving dish and put the veggies on individual tooth picks and dip that way.

Spinach Dip

1 pkg. 10 oz. frozen spinach, drained and thawed
1 ½ cups sour cream
1 cup Mayo (not Miracle Whip)
1 pkg. vegetable soup mix (dry)
1 (8oz.) can water chestnuts, drained and chopped

Blend all of the ingredients well. Put in covered container and chill.

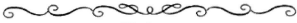

Notes:
Again... Use vegetables to dip. Spread on any deli meat and roll up.

Basic Dill Dip

      1 cup sour cream
      1 cup Mayo (not Miracle Whip)
      3 tsp. dill weed
      1 tsp. season salt
      2 Tbsp. minced onions
      2 Tbsp. dried parsley flakes

Mix well and chill.

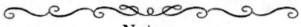

Notes:

If you thin this dip out with a little cream, it is awesome on a cheese omelet. Or, after the dip is thinned out a little with some cream, you can add it to your eggs before they are made into an omelet or scrambled! These are so yummy!

Did you know...? That if you spray the inside of a measuring cup with a non-stick spray before measuring out sticky ingredients, they will slide right out of the cup and clean up will be a breeze! (Peanut butter! Butter! Shortening!)

Miss Kelle's Three Cheese Dip

1 ½ cups diced American cheese
1 ½ cups cream
1 Tbsp. Worcestershire sauce
1 Tbsp. flour
1 tsp. dry or prepared mustard, if you like it
¾ cup cheddar cheese, shredded
¾ cup Swiss cheese, shredded
2 tsp. bottled hot sauce
¼ tsp. cayenne pepper

Sprinkle the flour on top of the cheese. Mix well. Add all of the other ingredients and cook over low heat, stirring constantly to prevent the cheese from sticking, until all the cheese is melted. Serve immediately. Dip vegetables or meatballs.

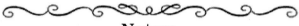

Notes:

For variation: you can add ½ cup red, orange, yellow or green pepper, diced. Add them all or add just one. It gives the sauce some color and depth. And once again... I don't think I have to tell you what this is like on an omelet or on the inside of the omelet with one of the sauces on the top. If you are going for the omelet, try a few bacon bits too! How about some diced ham or turkey...

Wait! We can't go anywhere without Miss Kelle's Three Cheese Dip. She says that too many people like to dip their veggies in cheese like a fondue! This is excellent!

I think this gives us enough variety to get started on our adventure. Remember, in no time you should be able to come up with your own creative recipes. Make sure you do try creating your own. The whole idea here is that we never want to get bored, right? You need to be able to do this on your own.

TIP: Anything no or low carb that you can put on a tooth pick is worthy of a test plunge into the sauces and dips! Who knows, you might find you like something you never before thought you would like! Believe me, it all helps.

TIP: Most cheeses should be served at room temperature to maximize their flavors.

Remember... never toil over which seed in the "garden of life" you have been given. Give it a lot of fertilizer and tend to it with loving care... for every seed in the garden produces that in which it was intended to produce. Every seed being just as important as the next, to the "master of the garden".

READY FOR APPETIZERS

When someone says appetizer to me, I have always looked at them as a pre-meal warm up, haven't you? A little preview of what is to come? A little something to start the engine? This is our nature my friends, (most of us any way). Is that you sitting there right now thinking to yourself, I'm sure glad she is not talking about me? You know I'm not talking about you. I'm talking about the rest of us. I wouldn't drag you into this. Really!

WHY did it take me the better part of my life to figure out that the appetizer SHOULD have been the WHOLE meal? But, as I've always said, let the good times roll! Let's face it, we live in a super-sized, super-super sized society. We keep paying more and more, for less and less nutrition in our food today, unless you are eating in some restaurants, per say. I just read an article in our local paper the other day that said, (hang on to your seats!) that the average steak in a steak house today is an 8-10 person serving size in just one steak! I didn't know whether to laugh or cry! I guess that sort of makes my Hubby a party unto himself! I don't know if you know any one like this yourself but, "all you can eat prime rib?" Are we there yet? Bring on the beef!

Have you ever been to France? Can you even imagine getting anything super-sized in France? The first time I saw a plate of French cuisine, I'm not kidding, I thought it was a sample! What is that? A taste test? How could anyone live on THAT I thought! I have learned a little something since those days, and that little something has brought me a long way in my thinking and living to present day.

I think those French people know a little bit about what they are doing after all! Smaller portions, larger FLAVOR and NUTRITION! Why? Because it does not take as much food to satisfy you. As it goes, it all comes back to nutrition, flavor and presentation. It fills all the senses, making us feel much more satisfied in the end of it all. Makes sense to me, how about you? What a concept! And that brings us exactly to the point of what this book is about.

Suppose we start to change our thinking just a little bit at this point? Why not try using an appetizer as a main course and just see what happens. You don't have to do it all the time, but just try it. We have nothing to lose do we? (Oh yes! I think I found it!) We can use one appetizer as the main course or we can combine two, three or more. You know, the ones we make at home? Eat alone or have a few friends over and throw a little party.

We are going to learn to plan and make what we feel to be some awesome appetizers. You can use them for just that, appetizers or a main meal. You "guys", these are great for football games, card parties or whatever you like to do. Have appetizers... will travel.

The TRICK is in finding something jazzy and delish! Something worth giving up those pizzas, chips, breadsticks and frosted doughnut holes for, right?

It's time now, to come along with me to the Cottage House Kitchen, where we just might be able to introduce you to some pretty exciting, mouth-watering party-time appetizers. Our hope is that you will like them so well that you will continue to want to eat them forever. That is one little step at a time towards our success!

If you like them, try to get as many appetizers made up ahead of time as possible. You never know when you are going to be starving, on the run, or having unexpected guests stopping over. Remember, if you don't have to think about it, chances are, you will get into a lot less trouble! Let's go for success! We CAN do it! And not only that, it will be fun!

The Latch Hook Inn's Fabulous Meatballs for Dipping

1 ½ lbs. ground pork
¼ cup chopped green onion
2 Tbsp. Teriyaki sauce
1/3 cup bacon bits
½ cup Parmesan cheese
2 tsp. minced garlic
1 egg
coarse salt and cracked pepper

Mix all ingredients. Form into walnut sized balls and sauté in frying pan until cooked thoroughly but not over cooked. Stir frequently to prevent the meatballs from sticking to the pan. Serve warm with any of the Cottage House sauces or dips. Throw a few in a food container and take some to work for snacks or lunch. The kids might like them in their lunch also.

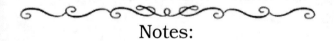

Notes:

Remember... if we were as good to ourselves as we are to our friends, they might not want to stick around very long. We deserve some nice things too. Let's be good to ourselves!

TIP: These meatballs can be chopped up and used to make omelets. Add them to scrambled eggs and top with a sauce.

Did you know... that no matter how wilted your celery is, all you have to do is soak it in a cold water bath and it will spring right back to life? This works well with many vegetables.

Sunny Creek's Firehouse Meatballs

1 ½ lb. ground beef
1/3 cup minced onion
2 Tbsp. habanera or other hot sauce
1 small jalapeño or pepper of choice, chopped fine
1 tsp. minced garlic
½ cup Parmesan cheese, grated
1egg
a few red pepper flakes, optional
coarse salt and cracked pepper

Mix well. Sauté in frying pan until cooked thoroughly but not over done. Stir frequently to keep meatballs from sticking to pan. Insert tooth pick into each meatball and serve warm with any Cottage House sauce or dip.

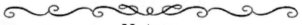

Notes:

These meatballs can be broken up and used in any omelet. Mix them into scrambled eggs and add a cheese sauce on top. These are great for tail-gaiting, and parties! Refrigerate and make plenty of them up ahead of time so that you will have them on hand for the week. These are a fabulous protein boost if you are on the go. If you eat them for breakfast... I'm sure they'll wake you up!

Did you know...? How to make the perfect hard-boiled egg? Take a dozen eggs, put them carefully into a pan. Cover them with tap water, add a tablespoon or two of white vinegar and salt the water. Bring them up just to a point where they start to boil... but do not let them boil. Turn off heat and cover with a lid. Leave them sit in the covered pan for 30 minutes. Drain them and submerge them in cold water. When they are cooled down, place them back into the egg containers and refrigerate. Now you have the perfect egg.

Milford Pond's Breakfast or Anytime Dipping Balls

1 ½ lbs. seasoned breakfast sausage, bulk
1/3 cup minced onion
½ cup chopped green olives
1 tsp. minced garlic
1 egg, slightly beaten
1/3 cup bacon bits
½ cup Parmesan cheese
1 Tbsp. cream

Mix well. Shape into balls the size of walnuts and sauté in frying pan until cooked thoroughly but not over done. Stir frequently to prevent the meatballs from sticking to the pan. Insert a tooth pick into each meatball and serve warm with dipping sauce.

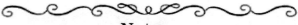

Notes:

The cheese sauces go especially well with these meatballs. Make plenty up ahead of time so that you have them on hand. Planning ahead prevents a crisis later on when you are hungry! These can also be chopped up and used in omelets or scrambled eggs with a cheese sauce on top.

Food is one situation where it's okay to try to re-invent the wheel!

If you have the time on a Saturday or Sunday morning to spend with your loved ones for brunch, why not take out your prettiest tablecloth, your nicest dishes, best flatware and glasses and set a beautiful table! Add a little bouquet of bright fresh flowers and a candle and really dazzle them. That is something that is so nice that they will probably always remember it. If you are alone, invite a friend or neighbor over and share the same thing with them. I had a friend who did that for me once, for no reason! It made me feel so good that I will never forget it!

Did you ever call someone up just to tell them that you love them and hang up the phone right after? It's very dramatic and I don't know of a person that would not smile for hours after that!

Saturday Night Bell Pepper Nachos

1 green bell pepper, cut into chunks
1 red bell pepper, cut into chunks
1 yellow bell pepper, cut into chunks
1 orange bell pepper, cut into chunks
sliced black olives
sliced green olives
real bacon bits
shredded cheese, any kind or a combination

Arrange peppers skin side down on a heat-proof platter. Sprinkle with olives and bacon bits, making sure to get them in the centers of the peppers. Top liberally with any shredded cheese you like or a combination of cheese. Place in the broiler for about three minutes or until the cheese is melted and the veggies are a little crisped.

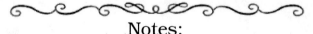

Notes:
While these vegetables have some carbohydrates in them, they have a lot of nutritional value. They are not empty carbs. I personally do not pay much attention to the carbs in these veggies because the alternative in nachos is not an option. I think that given a chance, you will also come to like these better and they scream Antioxidants! These are delish! They are complex carbs.

Experiment with your cheeses. Don't get stuck in a rut! There are tons of hard cheeses out there that are packed with flavor! Try not to use processed cheese, it's just not as good as the real deal. Some of our favorites are Brie, Jarlsberg, Fontina, Havarti, Gouda, and Gorgonzola. You'll see! The list goes on and on! If you are going to experience cheese, get the most flavor you can. Check them out! Expand your senses because remember now, you are going to become your own personal chef!

MoJo's Hot n' Spicy Chicken Wings

24 chicken wings or drummies
½ tsp. five spice
½ cup bottled hot sauce
½ tsp. ground cumin
1 bottle chili sauce
½ tsp. coarse salt
½ tsp. liquid smoke
½ cup orange juice
¼ tsp. cracked pepper

First, heat oil in deep fryer to 375 degrees. Deep fry plain wings for 5-7 minutes or until lightly browned. Drain.

Next, put all the hot sauce ingredients in a sauce pan. Bring to a simmer, stirring occasionally. Remove from heat. Transfer sauce to a large bowl. Add deep fried chicken wings and coat them really well.

Then, heat oven to 375 degrees. Line a jelly roll pan with foil and spray with non-stick spray. Transfer the wings to the pan in a single layer. Bake 10-15 minutes, making sure not to burn them. Transfer to serving platter. Add a bowl of MoJo's chunky cheese dip to center of platter.

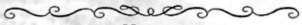

Notes:
Did someone say awesome? You be the judge! We can't leave these alone! This is a party on a platter!

MoJo's Chunky Cheese Dip

1 cup buttermilk
1 Tbsp. lemon juice
2 cups Mayo (not Miracle Whip)
1-2 tsp. bottled hot sauce
1 cup sour cream
2 tsp. Worcestershire sauce
½ cup minced onion
1 cup crumbled Blue Cheese
1 Tbsp. dried parsley
coarse salt and pepper
½ cup Parmesan cheese
garlic powder to taste

Mix well and refrigerate for several hours or overnight if you can. If you do not like Blue Cheese you can omit the cheese. This is too good to be to be true!

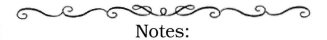

Notes:

Sonje's Bacon Wrapped Water chestnuts

2 can whole water chestnuts
¾ cup water
1 Tbsp. soy sauce
1 Tbsp. oil
2 Tbsp. Teriyaki sauce
½ tsp. garlic powder
1 lb. bacon

Cut the whole slab of bacon into thirds. Wrap each water chestnut with one third piece of bacon and secure with a tooth pick. Place on jelly roll pan and broil 5-10 minutes or until bacon is browned. Mix the rest of the ingredients together and drizzle over the water chestnuts and bake at 350 degrees for 25 minutes, turning occasionally.

Serve warm, cold, alone or with a dipping sauce.

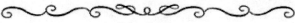

Notes:
Great to take to work as a snack. Try to have plenty on hand so that you can nibble.

Did you know...? That if you rub Peppermint Essential Oil on your temples (not too close to your eyes, because it is strong), on the back of your neck and forehead, it will do a good job of clearing out your head. It gets rid of a lot of headaches and really relaxes you. I highly recommend that you try it. Pamper yourself!

TIP: When you bottom out at work and you can't keep your eyes open, put a couple of drops of Peppermint, Grapefruit, Citrus or Lemon Essential Oil under your nose. Take a few deep breaths and you should be right back in the ball game. If not, repeat until you are. What a pick-me-up!

Back Alley Smoked Sausage Kabobs

6 smoked sausage links (ring style works also)
1 lb. of baby bella or button mushrooms
2 or 3 green peppers, cut into wedges
1 container of cherry tomatoes
2-3 onions, cut into small wedges
¼ cup Italian dressing
3 Tbsp. Teriyaki sauce
soaked bamboo skewers or regular skewers

Slice sausages into 1 inch chunks. Start alternating all the ingredients onto the skewers until you reach the top of the skewer. Repeat until you have the desired number of skewers.

Next, mix Italian dressing and Teriyaki sauce in large container with lid. Then add the skewers and marinate until needed, making sure to rotate the skewers so that they all get coated. BBQ on grill or broil them!

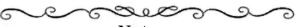

Notes:

You can make these up ahead of time and when you are ready to cook them, you can either broil them in the broiler or barbeque them on the grill. These are very tasty.

-- Again... the vegetables have some carbs in them. I don't really worry about them because they are packed with nutrition and Antioxidants. If you are going carb-less then leave them out.

These kabobs are fantastic for picnics or cooking out in the back yard. Actually... these are a meal on a skewer!

Cottage Pantry Blue Ribbon Deviled Eggs

12 eggs, hard boiled (the perfect boiled egg?)
¼-½ cup Mayo (not Miracle Whip)
2 tsp. mustard
4 oz. soft cream cheese
½ packet dry Italian dressing mix
¼ cup baby shrimp (cooked, patted dry and diced)
1-2 tsp. dried parsley flakes
1 Tbsp. cream
paprika
extra whole baby shrimp, cooked and patted dry

First, you will want to hard-boil the eggs and let them cool completely. Shell the eggs and cut them in half, length wise, and remove the yolks in the same manner you would to de-pit an avocado. Mash the egg yolks in a bowl. Add the cream cheese and blend well. Add the rest of the ingredients except the whole shrimp and paprika.

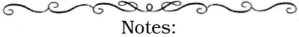

Notes:
Continues...

... Cottage Pantry Blue Ribbon Deviled Eggs (Cont'd)

Next... you will want to pipe the yolk mixture into the hole in the egg whites. You can use a spoon, but it looks a lot nicer if you take the time to use a pastry bag. If you do not have a pastry bag, don't panic! All you have to do is take a food storage bag, fill with yolk mixture, push it all to one corner, squeeze all the air out of the bag, twist the top closed tightly, and snip the corner of the bag off. Now you will be able to squeeze the mixture right into the egg white. Anyone can do it! You will be able to get a little fancy with the distribution of your egg yolk mixture into the egg whites in no time.

Finally, you want to put a baby shrimp on top of the egg yolk mixture on each egg and perhaps a slice of black or green olive. Sprinkle with paprika.

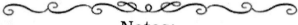

Notes:
To keep your eggs from sliding around on the plate, lay down some lettuce of your choice. Lay the eggs on top of the lettuce.

Roscoe's Stuffed Mushroom Mania

10-12 large mushrooms, like portabella
1 cup ricotta cheese
½ cup mozzarella cheese
½ cup cheddar cheese
1 cup Parmesan cheese, reserve half of it
4 Tbsp. crumbled bacon
4 Tbsp. pesto sauce
olive oil

First, preheat oven to 375 degrees.

Next, wash mushrooms, pat dry, remove stems and hollow out caps. Brush inside and out with olive oil. Mix remaining ingredients, reserving the ½ cup Parmesan cheese. Stuff the mushroom caps and sprinkle with remaining cheese. If you need more cheese, put more on!

Finally, place mushroom caps in small baking dish and bake in preheated oven for 20-25 minutes or until brown and crusty on top.

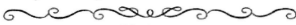

Notes:
What is life without stuffed mushrooms? They just seem to be everywhere and this looks like a good place to have them too.

TIP: you could mix one ounce of Marsala wine and one once of oil together (whisk to emulsify) and drizzle over the mushroom caps before you bake them.   Arrange mushroom caps on nice serving platter lined with finely shredded lettuce.   Garnish with lemon wedges in case you would like to drizzle lemon juice over the mushrooms.

You can also use prepared cellophane noodles to line your plate.   Put a few drops of food coloring in the water when you soak them.   Make sure to rinse!

Castle Cove Chicken Terrine

1½ lbs. uncooked cubed chicken breasts
1 pkg. dry Italian dressing mix
2 Tbsp. chopped scallions
¼ cup dried parsley flakes
1 tsp. dried tarragon leaves
½ tsp. coarse salt
¼ tsp. cracked pepper
2 egg whites
1 whole red bell pepper, diced very fine
1 sm. can Mandarin oranges, patted dry, & diced
extra whole Mandarin oranges
1½ Tbsp. olive oil

Recipe Continues...

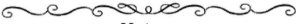

Notes:

If you are looking for something a little more elegant to serve at a luncheon, wedding shower or dinner party, this is very tasty and it makes a great presentation on the table. We like to use a silver serving tray lined with some pretty colored lettuce of your choice. Simply set the terrine on top of the lettuce and garnish with dried parsley leaves and orange sections arranged around sides of terrine. Cut a couple of slices to start the terrine and you are good to go. Add some red or green grapes to garnish to really get fancy.

...Castle Cove Chicken Terrine (Cont'd)

First, heat oven to 350 degrees.

Next, line loaf pan (8 ½ x 4 ½ x 2 ½) with foil. Spray the foil with non-stick spray and sprinkle with parsley liberally.

Then trim fat from chicken if necessary. Cut chicken into one inch pieces. Place chicken in food processor and pulse until coarsely ground. Add remaining ingredients except red bell pepper and Mandarin oranges, cover and process until smooth. Now add red bell pepper and Mandarin oranges into the chicken mixture. Spread in pan.

Cover tightly with aluminum foil and bake for one hour.

Remove foil and continue to bake another 30 minutes.

Remove from oven, re-cover with foil and let stand one hour.

Finally, refrigerate at least 3 hours but no longer than 48 hours. When ready to serve, invert onto platter and garnish.

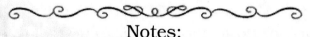

Notes:

Here is another appetizer, one more for the road. We need all the help we can get! This is made with the chicken terrine and we have found that it is great served at a party or football game.

What you do here is combine the great taste of the Castle Cove Chicken Terrine with a simple to make salsa. Takes care of any left-overs you might have! Here is the salsa recipe, as follows... Mad Man Marco's Simple Salsa!

Mad Man Marco's Simple Salsa

2 roma tomatoes, diced
½-1 can Mandarin oranges, chopped
1 small red bell pepper, diced
¼ cup coarsely chopped cilantro
2 green onions, chopped fine
1-2 fresh jalapeños, seeded and minced
2 Tbsp. fresh lime juice
1 tsp. minced garlic
1-2 Tbsp. vegetable oil
coarse salt

First, mix all ingredients in small bowl.

Next, let stand covered at room temperature for 1-2 hours to blend flavors.

Then, slice the chicken terrine into slices and arrange on a serving platter lined with lettuce. Dabble the salsa over the pieces. If you don't have the time to make the salsa, you could use the store bought kind, but it won't taste the same! This is good salsa.

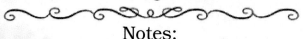

Notes:

Roddy's Smoked Sausage and Veggie Hot Pockets

1 lb. smoked sausage, cut into one inch pieces
1 small butternut squash, peeled & cut into 1" pieces
1 red bell pepper, seeded & cut into 1" pieces
1 cup cauliflower florets, smaller pieces
1 cup Monterey Jack cheese, shredded
any of the herbed butters in this book
coarse salt and cracked black pepper

If you do not have the herbed butters, use regular butter and dried herbs instead.

First, cut 6 18x12 inch pieces of heavy duty foil.
Next, in bowl, combine all of the ingredients and mix.
Place mixture onto each sheet of foil. Top with herbed butter, or regular butter and dried herbs.
Wrap each packet securely using double fold seals, allowing room for expansion.
Lastly, bake in 350 degree oven for 20-30 minutes or until vegetables are done to desired crispness.

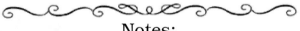

Notes:
These are huge on flavor and can be done up ahead of time. All you have to do when you need them is pop them in the oven or put them on the grill. Great for picnics or dinner at home.

Mario's Mushroom Fantasy

2 lbs. sliced or whole mushrooms, any variety
4 Tbsp. butter
1 tsp. minced garlic
2 Tbsp. good white wine
1 tsp. dried sweet basil
½ cup Parmesan cheese
coarse salt and cracked black pepper, or season salt

First, melt butter in frying pan. Add everything except the Parmesan cheese. Sauté until liquid is mostly reduced. Add a little more butter and stir well. Remove from heat and transfer to serving dish.

Sprinkle with Parmesan cheese and a little dried parsley flakes and dig in!

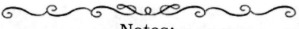

Notes:

If you are a mushroom lover... this one is for you. And irresistible it is! This is just an all around great appetizer or side dish. Use a variety of mushrooms together!

Pepperoni Chips

If you'd like something other than veggies or pork rinds to dip or snack on, try this. Go to the store or the butcher and get a large roll of pepperoni, about 3 inches in diameter if possible and have it sliced rather thin. If you can't do that, just by the pre-sliced in the package.

Place a couple of layers of paper towel on a microwave-safe plate. Place slices of pepperoni in a single layer on the plate. Microwave approximately 2 minutes until crisp but not burned. As all microwaves have different watts, check to make sure you do not burn them. Continue process until all of your pepperoni is cooked. These little slices are great just to snack on and they taste like bacon. Try dipping them or crunch them up and use like you would use bacon bits.

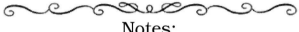

Notes:

You can make these up ahead of time and have a bunch of them on hand.

Here are a couple more things we thought you might like to try having some fun with.

Cheese Taco Shell

On microwave-safe plate, spray with non-stick spray. Add a layer of shredded Cheddar cheese approximately 8-9 inches in diameter. Microwave until crispy but not burned. Remove from microwave and quickly shape into the form of a taco shell. Do it while it is hot. These make a great no-carb taco shell. Now you can enjoy your tacos with very few carbs if any.

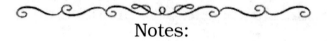

Notes:

Tip: All of the omelets that are in this book were made in the microwave, approx. 1000 watts. Cooking times may vary because all microwaves are different. Watch and adjust cooking times. Any of the omelets that are in this book can also be made in a skillet on the stove as well. We just happen to feel it's a snap in the microwave... no pan to clean. It doesn't turn brown like it does from frying either. (unless you happen to like the crispy brown on the exterior of the omelet). It's all about what you like. I personally feel that the omelets turn out moister and smoother in the microwave. Always use the freshest eggs possible for best results!

ABOUT BREAKFAST

This is where I hope to come to a meeting of the minds. If you are like me and a few hundred thousand other people... breakfast? Who me? Not since I lived at home with my mother!

Friends, I hate to tell you what you already know, but breakfast IS your gas station! We need to fuel up right off the bat in the morning! The reason for this is not entirely to fill the hole in your stomach, it's as much about giving your body something to run on! The worse that can happen if you do not put fuel in your car is that it just plain won't run! Our bodies seem to be a little more forgiving than our automobiles, but over the long run, we pay for it in many different ways, and we know it!

When I ask people why they don't eat breakfast in the morning, the most common answer I get is, "I have a hard enough time just getting to work on time, let alone breakfast. I usually pick something up on the way". And I have then asked, "If you had something really tasty and satisfying already made up in the refrigerator to just grab and eat on the run, would you?" Well, in almost every case the answer has been yes, sure, probably and a few more like wise. My guess is that if you ate that good stuff from the refrigerator on your way out the door in the morning, you probably wouldn't even feel like stopping for that jelly doughnut by the time you got to the quickie mart. Never have an empty stomach because this is exactly where we lose our good judgment and get right into trouble!

Well friends, wouldn't it be nice if we could all have our own personal chef? You know, the kind the stars have? Wouldn't it be nice if all of our meals and snacks were precisely thought out and made up ahead of time for us? Presented to us on a fancy silver platter, the kind fit for a king? I think just about any body could stick with it in that case. To me, that's a no-brainer!

Unfortunately, we may not have our own personal chef, but we are going to become our own personal chef! I hear the job security stands second to none and it's really affordable. With a little luck, this chef won't be walking out on the job any time soon! We can do this! I'm going to show you a few tricks of the trade and it's not going to cost you a million dollars a year, just a little of your time. And the beauty of the whole thing is that the time you give up now, will save you a lot of time in the long run. It will also save you a lot of future judgment and eating disasters. How good does this get?

Remember now, we are on an adventure! We are going to make this fun! Work with me here!

If you have your appetizers, sauces, dips and vegetables made up ahead of time, this covers all breakfasts, snacks at home, snacks at work, kid's snacks or lunches and even loved-one's football party on the weekend! See what I mean about saving time? It's not hard! You can do it!

TIP: When it comes to counting the carbs in vegetables and fruit, if you are going for the absolute no carb thing then don't eat them. I personally eat them and I always will. I believe that they are packed with the vitamins, minerals and Antioxidants our bodies desperately need. My thought on this... I have never seen anyone become obese from eating too much broccoli or too many apples have you? You make your own decision on this one.

* Vegetables are complex carbohydrates.

Remember... if we were as good to our friends as we are to ourselves, they probably wouldn't stick around very long!

We are going to be talking about two kinds of breakfasts... The "No-time breakfast", and the "Have-time breakfast".   I hope this will cover the whole area of breakfast, leaving no openings to knock us off the track!

The "No-time breakfast" is obviously when you don't have time to prepare anything. This is the one that sets us up for disaster! Planning ahead can save the day! Here are some suggestions.

Start with appetizers. Any of the appetizers in this book can be used for breakfast as well as snacks or even meals. If we've done our job right we should have plenty of these made up ahead of time. Just grab and go. So, take one night, say Monday and make and make and make these appetizers.

Make a lot of deviled eggs and store them in a covered container in the refrigerator. Grab as needed. Fry up a lot of bacon and sausage or ham ahead of time and store in a covered container in the refrigerator. Grab a couple of pieces, warm in the microwave. Grab some deviled eggs and you have your bacon and egg breakfast. Done! Delish! Boil a dozen eggs for hard-boiled eggs to have on hand. Fry up a bunch of sausage or turkey patties, store in a covered container in the refrigerator. Smoked or polish sausage is great to have on hand. Cube up a bunch of different hard cheeses and store in baggies... instant breakfast or snack on the go. Kids love the cheese! The meatballs in the appetizer section of this book are so good, we eat them for breakfast all the time. Eat them with scrambled eggs which you can also make up ahead of time. Just warm and go!

Remember, breakfast is quintessential! It fires up the body furnace for the whole day's burning. The earlier you get started, the more you can burn. Once the momentum starts, it just keeps rolling. Don't waste a half a day because you by-passed breakfast for those jelly doughnuts!

And now for the "Have-time breakfast"

Do not just indulge in a "Have-time breakfast". Take time to really enjoy it with family or friends. Make it a celebration! Use your prettiest tablecloth, your nicest dish set, your best flatware and glassware. Add a bouquet of bright fresh flowers to the table. Light a candle and make it a total experience for everyone. Make it warm. Make it a happy occasion and your loved ones will never forget it. This is how you create memories!

The following recipes are going to be good ole' sit down, warm the tummy comfort food. Elegant enough to serve at a fancy brunch or just a regular breakfast.

Please do not think that the following recipes are just for breakfast. All of these recipes can be used any time or anywhere. Don't be afraid to experiment. Remember, the larger your meal repertoire, the larger your chance for success!

LET'S TALK ABOUT OMELETS A LITTLE BIT

We at the Cottage House do not feel that omelets are just for breakfast anymore. In this section, we are going to call them egg wraps. These egg wraps are so versatile that you can have them for any meal. I believe that these egg wraps are so wonderful, they even make elegant dinner fare.

As we talked about earlier, if we would like to succeed in a life time eating plan, we have to make the very most out of every meal.

Feeling of course that the omelet has been totally under-rated, I felt the need to take a closer look at what could be done to bring them up to speed. Why DON'T people make or order them for dinner more often... I thought to myself! Could it be that the good old ham and cheese omelet might be getting a little tired? Don't get me wrong, I like a ham and cheese omelet just as well as the next person, but where is the kick? Sorry my friends, this is so like me and my compulsive nature. I have to throw everything over the edge or I'm just not happy! You know... even when I go to a furniture store to buy an item, I will either have changed something about it or added something to it by the time I get it home. I don't know why I do this, I just do.

In the following pages, we are going to give you some eggie choices that we hope will put you well on your way to enjoying and even craving these fantastic, anytime of the day, egg presentations, instead of that potato or pasta dish.

Come along with us now, as we introduce you to the stars of the show... a little bit of egg heaven!

TIP: Just for fun... If you would like a new way to present your deviled eggs, take a platter, line the platter with a dark leafy lettuce and then add a layer of prepared cellophane noodles, not quite to the edge of the platter. Arrange the deviled eggs on top of the noodles and garnish with some fresh herbs and Mandarin orange sections. Color the noodles by adding food coloring to the water and soaking them. Rinse and decorate. Green works well with deviled eggs. Use your imagination!

Let's take a moment... on the subject of Hollandaise and Béarnaise sauces, since we will be using them quite a bit.

These are two great sauces that you can use on a lot of different dishes. Let's make them a little handy so that you can refer to them easily. Take advantage of these sauces and try them on a variety of things yourself! They are great on vegetables as well.

I'm In Paradise for the Hollandaise Sauce

3 egg yolks
1 cup sweet cream butter
½ tsp salt
1 Tbsp. lemon juice
1 Tbsp. heavy cream
dash cayenne pepper

Place egg yolks, salt, cayenne pepper and cream in a food processor or blender. Blend for a few seconds on high speed until you have a smooth frothy mixture. Set aside.

Melt butter in a small pan over low heat being careful not to brown or burn the butter.

With the food processor or blender at high speed, start adding the hot butter in a thin steady stream. As butter is added, the sauce will thicken. When half the butter has been added, add lemon juice and continue blending until all the butter has been used in the sauce.

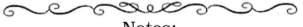

Notes:

It is desirable to use the home-made Hollandaise sauce. There are no carbs... if you are going to use the packaged variety... just make sure to check the carb count.

To make a Béarnaise sauce... all you really have to do is add some tarragon vinegar and some dried tarragon leaves to the Hollandaise sauce. You may also add a little wine if you like for more flavor. Experiment a little! There are many sauces that you can work with for all of these recipes, this is the fun part, you just need to decide what you like.

Sunday Morning Mimosa Wrap

2 eggs
2 Tbsp. sour cream
½ cup ricotta cheese
½ cup shredded Swiss cheese
½ cup fresh chopped spinach
1 Tbsp. real bacon bits
1 can (4 oz.) Mandarin oranges, drained, diced
Hollandaise sauce (our no carb recipe)
coarse salt and cracked black pepper

First, spray a dinner plate with a non-stick spray. Next, combine ricotta cheese, Swiss cheese, spinach, bacon bits and ½ of the diced oranges (reserving the rest as a garnish).

Prepare Hollandaise sauce and have that ready.

Recipe Continues...

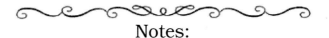

Notes:

...Sunday Morning Mimosa Wrap (Cont'd)

Beat eggs and sour cream until fluffy. Pour onto prepared plate and microwave 2 minutes or until the center is set. Remove from microwave.

Add a layer of filling down the middle to the ends of the omelet, making sure you leave enough room to roll it up.

Next... fold front over middle and middle over back to form a roll. Top with Hollandaise, oranges and parsley flakes. Microwave another 30 seconds or so until heated through. If you want to live dangerously, serve with a Mimosa Cocktail. Did I say that? Save up some carbs?

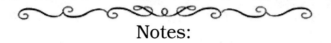

Notes:

Shrimp Ala Barbie Egg Wrap

2 eggs
2 Tbsp. sour cream
½ cup cooked baby shrimp
zest of one lemon or lime
¼ cup chopped roma tomatoes
1 Tbsp. green onion, chopped
½ cup Monterey Jack cheese, shredded
1½ cup prepared Béarnaise sauce
extra baby shrimp for garnish
extra shredded Monterey Jack cheese for garnish
extra chopped roma tomatoes for garnish
dried parsley flakes for garnish

Spray a dinner plate with a non-stick spray. Next, combine baby shrimp, lemon or lime zest, tomatoes, green onions, cheese and mix together and set aside.

Prepare Béarnaise sauce (preferably home-made)

Recipe continues...

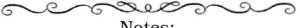

Notes:
If you are a shrimp lover... try this one. It's rich and elegant. This seems to be a favorite with family and friends... this is definitely something I can live with!

...Shrimp Ala Barbie Egg Wrap (Cont'd)

Beat eggs and sour cream until fluffy. Pour onto prepared plate and microwave two minutes or until eggs are set in the center. Remove from microwave.

Add a layer of filling down the middle to the ends of the omelet. Drizzle a liberal layer of Béarnaise sauce on top of the filling.

Fold the front over the middle and the middle over the back to form roll. Top with Béarnaise sauce, baby shrimp, cheese, chopped tomatoes and dried parsley flakes. Return to microwave oven for 30 or so seconds until heated through.

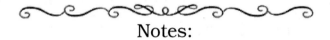

Notes:

Captain's Cove Cottage Club Wrap

2 eggs
2 Tbsp. sour cream
½ lb. deli turkey, ham or both
½ cup of diced roma tomatoes
¼ cup real bacon bits
¼ cup shredded Monterey Jack or Swiss cheese
sour cream or lite ranch dressing

First... spray a dinner plate with a non-stick spray.

Next... beat eggs and sour cream or dressing until fluffy. Pour onto prepared plate and microwave for two minutes or until center of eggs are set. Remove from microwave.

Next... add a layer of shredded meat, a layer of diced tomatoes, bacon bits, cheese and then a layer of sour cream or dressing down the middle of omelet making sure to leave enough room to be able to fold the omelet.

Next... fold the front over the middle, the middle over the back to form a roll. Drizzle sour cream or dressing over the top of omelet. Add a couple of diced tomatoes, bacon bits, shredded cheese and garnish with parsley flakes or green onions. Put back in the microwave for another 30 seconds or so, until it is heated through.

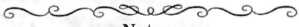

Notes:
If you love those club sandwiches, here is the next best thing to it. No bread... no guilt! In fact, these are richer than a club sandwich.

TIP: Never put salt in your eggs before they are cooked in a microwave because it will turn them rubbery.

Sunset Bay Monterey Wrap

Think about those sunsets on the beach. A romantic dinner for two and something light to eat before that evening stroll.

 2 eggs
 2 Tbsp. sour cream
 ½ cup cooked, shredded chicken
 ¼ cup shredded Monterey Jack cheese
 ¼ cup shredded cheddar cheese
 ½ cup chopped fresh spinach
 2 Tbsp. real bacon bits
 2 Tbsp. Raspberry Vinaigrette dressing
 Extra cheddar cheese for topping
 Extra Monterey Jack cheese for topping

First... Spray a dinner plate with a non-stick spray

Beat eggs and sour cream until fluffy. Pour onto prepared plate and microwave for two minutes or until center of eggs are set. Remove from microwave.

In a bowl combine shredded chicken, cheeses, spinach, and bacon bits and toss with the raspberry vinaigrette.

Down the center of the omelet to both ends add a layer of the chicken mixture, making sure to leave enough room to be able to fold the omelet like a roll up.

Fold the front over the middle, the middle over the back to form a roll. Top with extra cheese and microwave for another 30 seconds until heated through. Top with sour cream and fresh or dried parsley.

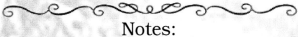

Notes:
The filling for these omelets should be able to fill two omelets in most of these recipes.

Ernesto's South of the Border Pulled Pork Wrap

2 eggs
2 Tbsp. sour cream
1 cup shredded or pulled cooked pork
1 small jalapeño pepper, de-seeded or not, and diced
¼ cup cheddar cheese, extra for topping
¼ cup shredded Monterey Jack cheese,
1 cup salsa
Sour cream
cilantro

Spray a dinner plate with a non-stick spray.

Beat eggs and sour cream until fluffy. Pour onto prepared plate and microwave for two minutes or until center of eggs are set. Remove from microwave.

In a bowl, combine the pork, jalapeño, cheeses and chopped cilantro to taste.

Down the center of omelet to both ends, add a layer of pork mixture. Drizzle Salsa on top of pork layer.

Fold the front over the middle, the middle over the back to form roll. Top with more cheeses and salsa. Microwave another 30 seconds or until heated through. Top with sour cream and cilantro to taste.

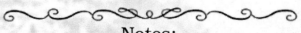

Notes:

You don't have to go to the Caribbean Riviera to enjoy this one... make it at home. It's an explosion of flavor. Party on a plate!

TIP: The fillings for all of these egg wraps can probably fill two or more wraps. The carbs in the salsa is minimal. Always use the freshest eggs possible for best omelets.

Chewey's Philly Egg Wrap

2 eggs
2 Tbsp. sour cream
1 cup of shredded deli beef (just pull beef apart)
¼ cup chopped green pepper
¼ cup diced onion
½ cup shredded Swiss or cheddar cheese
2 Tbsp. Italian dressing

Spray a dinner plate with a non-stick spray

Beat eggs and sour cream until fluffy. Pour onto prepared plate. Microwave for two minutes or until center of eggs are set. Remove from microwave.

In bowl, combine beef, green pepper, onion, cheese and Italian dressing and toss to coat.

Down the center and to the ends of omelet, add a layer of the meat mixture making sure to leave enough room to form roll when folded.

Fold the front over the middle and the middle over the back to form roll. Top with cheese, green peppers and onions if desired and put back in the microwave and cook for another 30 seconds until heated thoroughly. Top with sour cream if desired

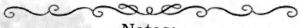

Notes:

This of course is a nice twist on the Philly Steak and Cheese. We think you will be pleasantly surprised, and now you don't have to give up those steak and cheese!

Hattie Mae's Sunday Morning Quiche

2 cups raw chicken breast, cut into pieces
1½ cups frozen broccoli florets
1½ cups sliced mushrooms
½ cup shredded cheddar cheese
1 cup heavy cream
½ cup milk
5 eggs
2-3 tsp. prepared mustard
1 cup shredded Swiss cheese
¼ - ½ tsp. cayenne pepper or hot sauce to taste
coarse salt and cracked black pepper
Parmesan cheese
10 inch pie plate sprayed with non-stick spray

First... spray the pie plate with the non-stick spray.

Next... sauté chicken, broccoli and mushrooms in some butter until chicken is cooked through and broccoli is tender. Do not over cook. Remove from heat, let cool a little and add Cheddar cheese. Pour into pie plate.

Next... in bowl, combine cream, milk, eggs, Mustard, cheese, salt, pepper and cayenne pepper. Pour over chicken and broccoli mixture. Sprinkle with Parmesan cheese. Bake in 375 degree oven... 45 minutes to 1 hour, until the center is set. Let cool for 10 minutes before cutting. (If you don't want to sauté chicken, you can use canned or already cooked).

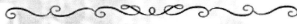

Notes:

Hattie Mae puts on a Sunday brunch fit for a king. When you taste this quiche you are going to say... "It's really rough eating like this, isn't it?" That's exactly what we say!

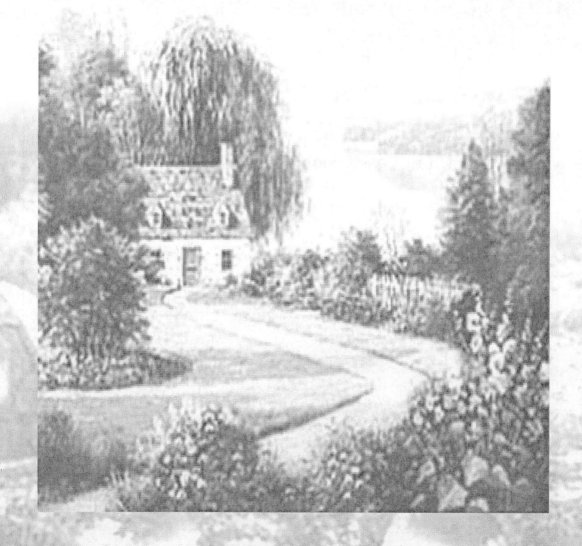

Captain Jack's Steamboat Brunch... "Club Quiche"

1½ cups cooked and diced turkey
1 cup bacon, cooked, drained and crumbled
1 cup roma tomatoes, seeded and diced
½ cup shredded cheddar cheese
1 cup cream
½ cup milk
1 cup shredded Swiss cheese
5 eggs
1 tsp. minced garlic
½ cup Parmesan cheese
coarse salt and cracked black pepper
sweet basil
10 inch pie plate sprayed with non-stick spray

First... spray the pie plate with non-stick spray.

Next... to pie plate add the turkey, bacon, tomatoes and cheddar cheese. Spread out evenly. Sprinkle with sweet basil.

Then... in bowl, combine the cream, milk, eggs, salt, pepper and garlic. Beat until smooth. Add Swiss cheese and mix well. Pour over turkey mixture. Top with Parmesan cheese.

Finally... bake in 375 degree oven... 45-60 minutes or until the center is set. Cool ten minutes before cutting. Cut in wedge, place on plate, sprinkle with parsley, garnish with a fresh flower bud. If you want to get fancy, add some Hollandaise sauce over the top of the quiche... why not?

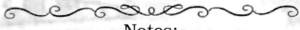

Notes:

Be a guest of the Captain's this morning... or at least you'll feel like royalty when you sit down to this rich and tasty brunch.

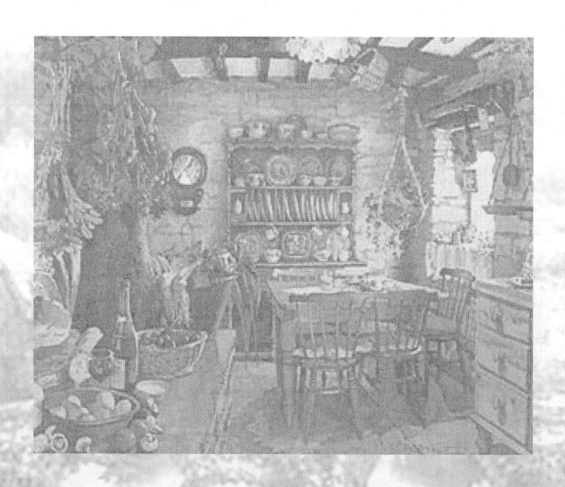

Tip: For recipes that call for cooked and cut up chicken, the trick is to buy the already made rotisserie chicken from the store.   De-bone, cut up and freeze to have on hand when you need them.   They are wonderfully seasoned to boot. We usually buy a few and freeze them.

Carolina Jerry's "Ole" Southern Eggs with Cheesy Country Gravy

5 Tbsp. butter
2 cups diced regular or honey ham
2 cups diced celery
2 cups fresh or canned mushrooms
10-12 eggs
2 ½ cups cream
¾ cup American cheese. Shredded or cubed
2 tsp. prepared mustard
salt, pepper and cayenne pepper

First... in a non-stick or well seasoned cast iron skillet, melt butter over low heat. Throw in the celery, ham, and mushrooms and sauté until tender.

Next... in bowl, combine eggs and ½ cup cream. Beat well. Scramble in separate pan and add to ham mixture. In saucepan, add two cups cream, American cheese, mustard, cayenne pepper or hot sauce and salt and pepper. Simmer on low heat until the sauce thickens to the consistency you like. Drizzle over eggs. Add more hot sauce if you like. Serve alone or with sausage patties.

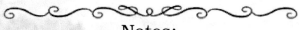

Notes:
There is something about this flavor combination that is right out of this world. This dish to us is totally tasty, satisfying, good old comfort food!

Milford Pond's Eggs Benedict

2 lbs. tasty seasoned breakfast sausage (bulk)
6-8 eggs, poached or sunny side up
½ cup roma tomatoes, chopped
1 or so cups Hollandaise sauce, prepared
sweet paprika

First... You will want to make 6-8 large sausage patties. They can be a good third pound each, or fourth pound... whatever you prefer. Fry the sausage patties and put on paper towel to drain. You can cover them and keep them warm in a low oven if you desire.

Next... Prepare the Hollandaise sauce so that it is ready. Add the chopped tomatoes to Hollandaise sauce. If you are using the packaged brand of Hollandaise sauce, check the Carb content on package.

Recipe Continues...

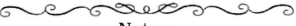

Notes:

Who says you can't have Eggs Benedict any more? Get a load of this! I think our version is even better than the restaurant deal. Tried and true... this is our all time favorite.

...Milford Pond's Eggs Benedict (Cont'd)

Next... You will want to make the eggs, any way you like them. We've tried them both ways and they are equally as good poached or sunny side up.

Next... Assemble the eggs benedict. On a plate, lay down a nice piece of lettuce. Place the sausage patty on top of the lettuce. Put the poached or sunny side up egg on top of the sausage patty and pour on the Hollandaise sauce. Sprinkle with paprika. Garnish the plate with a stem of green or red grapes. And of course... oranges always work well as a garnish too. You can substitute turkey sausage or ham for the breakfast sausage. This dish is delish!

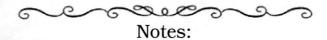

Notes:

Miss Sophie's Breakfast Platter

Got left-overs in the fridge? Things that didn't get eaten up all week? Here is a fabulous way to move them on... not to waste!

First... Take a large turkey platter and line it with some lettuce leaves. Try some that are pretty in color.

Next... Place on the platter what ever you have left over in the fridge. Add some Crème Fresh to it if you wish. Bacon strips, sausage patties, deviled eggs, left over appetizers. Any left-over quiche? Add that too! How about some cubed cheese?

You get the idea! Be creative... have a little buffet. This is the time to clean the left-overs out so that you can start fresh for the next week. Don't waste a thing. Add a few grape clumps if you don't mind a few extra carbs, they are loaded with vitamins anyway!

Remember... there are three kinds of people in this world... those who make things happen... those who watch what happened... and those who wonder what happened!

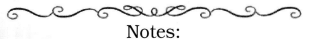

Notes:

DINNER SELECTIONS

From the Cottage House Kitchen comes a celebration of life, love and good food. Think about how you can enjoy a meal with someone you love. Home alone tonight? Call a friend! Deliver a meal to someone who can't get out of the house. Cook a meal for someone's Birthday or Anniversary. What a great gift to give. Deliver it to their home, you'll be surprised how quickly you forget about the day's troubles, you won't have time to think about them.

Do you love to cook but you don't have anyone to cook for? I don't know of too many people who would turn down a home cooked meal. Around here, we bake and feed the neighborhood, family and friends. If you have the passion... just do it! We have plenty of taste-testers around here just waiting for a free sample! I'll bet you would too!

Live, love, laugh and lighten up! Try to leave your problems behind for awhile.

You may not be eating muffins yourself, but wouldn't it be nice to bake some and take them to an elderly shut-in? How about a pan of brownies to the Widow next door?

It's a fact that when you do something nice for someone else, you feel better yourself.

Now come along with me and let's see what's coming out of the Cottage House Kitchen just for you!

Totally Outrageous Turkey Divan

2 (10oz.) pkgs. frozen broccoli florets (or fresh)
or mixed vegetables (carrots, broccoli and cauliflower)
2-3 turkey breasts, sautéed and chunked
1 cup heavy cream
½ cup sour cream
1 cup Mayo (not Miracle Whip)
1 Tbsp. lemon juice
1 tsp. curry powder
2 cups shredded cheddar cheese
sweet paprika
½ cup ground pork rinds, optional (for bread crumbs)
2 Tbsp. melted butter for ground pork rinds
salt and pepper

Spray a 9x13 casserole dish with non-stick spray.

Steam the vegetables until slightly tender but do not over cook.

Place the vegetables in the bottom of the casserole dish and spread out evenly.

Sauté the turkey pieces in butter until browned but not over cooked.

Recipe continues...

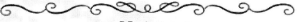

Notes:

This is an absolutely awesome dish... It tastes like a million bucks and it only has minimal carbs. The few carbs that will be in here are nutritious carbs and worth every bit of it. Totally satisfying! Remember, we are trying to eat things we can live with. No boredom or starvation please! Life is too short!

...Totally Outrageous Turkey Divan (Cont'd)

Put the turkey pieces over the vegetables, spreading out evenly.

Combine the heavy cream, sour cream and Mayo in bowl. Add the curry powder and lemon juice. Salt and pepper to taste.

Pour the sauce over the vegetables and turkey and top with the cheddar cheese.

Toss the ground pork rinds with the melted butter and sprinkle on top of the cheese if desired.

Bake in 350 degree oven around 30 minutes or until hot and bubbly. Sprinkle with paprika as garnish.

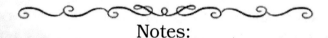

Notes:

Chicken Lombardi from The Blue Lagoon

4-6 boneless, skinless chicken breasts, thawed
1-2 lbs. fresh sliced mushrooms, any variety
1 cup shredded mozzarella cheese
1 cup Parmesan cheese
½ cup Marsala wine
½ cup chicken stock
coarse salt and cracked black pepper

Brown the chicken breasts in butter making sure not to over cook (if they are not done, that's all right because you will be finishing them off in the oven anyway).

Reserve the pan drippings from the chicken and add more butter to the pan. Add a little Marsala wine and all of the mushrooms. Sauté the mushrooms until the liquid is reduced.

Recipe Continues...

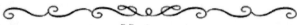

Notes:
This is a dish that is elegant enough for a candle light dinner. If that's not the case... munch it in front of the television. It's packed with flavor and so simple to make.

... Chicken Lombardi from the Blue Lagoon (Cont'd)

Put the chicken breasts in a 9x13 cake pan in a single layer. Spoon the mushrooms and any left over liquid over the chicken breasts.

In the same pan you used for the chicken, add some more butter (about 3 Tbsp.), the Marsala wine and the chicken stock. Simmer for about 10 minutes.

Pour the sauce over the chicken and bake 10-20 minutes at 375 degrees. Take out of the oven and sprinkle liberally with Parmesan cheese and top with mozzarella. Baste with a little of the juice from the pan and continue to bake until cheese is melted and bubbly.

Place chicken breast on a plate and drizzle with additional sauce from the pan. Add salt and pepper to taste. This is so good!

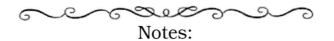

Notes:

No Problem Lady! Jamaican Pork Tenderloin

2 lb. pork tenderloin

marinade made of:
½ cup brown sugar
¾ cup orange juice
½ cup lime juice
2 Tbsp. minced garlic
1 tsp. salt
1 tsp. black pepper
½ tsp. allspice
1 tsp. ginger
1 tsp. grated orange peel
1 tsp. grated lime peel
3 Tbsp. olive oil

First... mix all the marinade ingredients together and blend thoroughly.

Next... score the tenderloin criss-cross on the top side.

Next... place tenderloin in a one gallon sized zip lock baggie. Add the marinade and seal very tightly.

Next... marinate at least 4 hours and preferably over night. Rotate periodically.   Recipe continues...

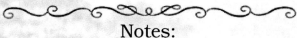

Notes:

Next... after it has marinated, in an oiled hot skillet, quickly sauté (brown) tenderloin to seal in the juices. Do not worry about cooking through because you are going to finish it off in the oven.

Next... transfer the tenderloin to a bake dish and spoon some of the marinade over the top of it. Bake 350 degrees ½ - 1 hour depending on size.

Next... return the pan with the marinade in it to the stove. You should have about a cup of sauce in the pan, if there is a lot more, discard. To the marinade add 1 cup of heavy cream and simmer over low heat until the sauce reduces and thickens. This could take several minutes... but it will reduce and thicken. When it reaches desired consistency, remove from stove.

Next... when the tenderloin is done baking and has rested for about 10 minutes... slice it on the diagonal, into half inch slices. Fan whatever portion size you desire onto a serving plate and drizzle the sauce over the top of the meat. Garnish with some lime wedges. Serve with some cubed cheese if you are really hungry.

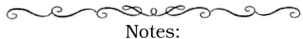

Notes:

TIP: As a side dish, try broiling or roasting a bunch of cherry or grape tomatoes in oil on a jelly roll pan. Sprinkle with dried sweet basil and Parmesan cheese. Add salt and pepper, and roast or broil until cheese is melted and tomatoes soften a little and are heated through. Yummy!

Uncle Nunzio's Italian Sausage Egg Bake

This is it! Uncle Nunzio's kitchen on Saturday evening. Lot's of people... lots of love! There just isn't a better dinner in anybody's neighborhood! Eggs aren't just for breakfast anymore! Ala Familia!

1 large serving platter
2 lbs. ring smoke sausage, cut in chunks on diagonal
4 Tbsp. butter
1 each, red, orange, yellow and green bell pepper
    seeded and cut into chunks
1 lb. fresh or canned mushrooms
1 lg. Onion, cut into chunks
1 ½ cups celery, chopped
1 ½ cups shredded cheddar cheese
10-12 eggs... 4 Tbsp. butter
1/3 cup sour cream
½ tsp. dried sweet basil or Italian seasoning
2 cups heavy cream
1 cup American cheese
2 tsp. prepared mustard
¼ tsp. cayenne pepper
2 tsp. bottled hot sauce

Recipe continues...

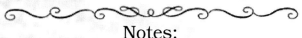

Notes:

First... slice sausage in half inch pieces on the diagonal and put in oiled or buttered hot skillet. Add the peppers, mushrooms and celery in large skillet. Cook down until it all starts to caramelize a little.

Next... combine eggs, cream and sweet basil or Italian seasoning. Whisk until fluffy. Pour egg mixture into a separate buttered skillet and cook eggs until they are scrambled but not over-cooked.

Next... add the cream, cheese, mustard, pepper and hot sauce in sauce pan. Simmer until thickened (about 10 minutes, the longer you cook it the thicker it will get) to the desired consistency. It should look rich, coat the back of the spoon, and look glossy smooth.

Next... combine the egg mixture with the sausage mixture and toss well to distribute everything.

Next... heap the whole sausage-egg mixture onto a large serving platter and drizzle lots of the cheese sauce over the whole thing! Garnish with fresh parsley and lots of orange sections. This dish is WELL worth the fuss!

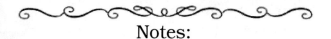

Notes:

Wild Willie's Patio Party Egg Bake

8 eggs
1 tsp. bake powder
salt and pepper to taste
3 cups shredded Monterey Jack cheese
1 ½ cups shredded cheddar cheese
1 cup cooked and crumbled bacon
1/3 cup sun-dried tomatoes, diced
4 Tbsp. chopped green olives
1 Tbsp. green onion, chopped
1/3 cup heavy cream

First... heat oven to 375 degrees. Spray a casserole dish with a non-stick spray.

Next... combine eggs and cream and beat until fluffy, around 5 minutes or so.

Next... add baking powder and salt, whisk together well and fold in cheeses, bacon, tomatoes, olives and table onions.

Next... pour into prepared casserole dish and bake 20-25 minutes. Sprinkle with extra cheese five minutes before removing from oven. Let stand for 10 minutes before serving.

Top with Hollandaise sauce, cheese sauce or a dollop of sour cream. Garnish with dried parsley and sweet paprika or more green onion.

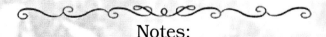

Notes:

Remember... for some people... no explanation is necessary at all... and for some... no explanation will suffice.

Crawdaddy's Crustacean Creation with Creamy Creole Sauce

9 inch pie plate sprayed with non-stick spray
1 ½ cups cooked baby shrimp, rinsed and patted dry
1 cup frozen broccoli, cooked, drained, not over done
½ cup celery
¼ cup carrot
¼ cup green onion, chopped
1 tsp. minced garlic
1 cup cream
2 tsp. bottled hot sauce
½ cup milk
¼ tsp. cayenne pepper
5 eggs
½ tsp. dill weed
1 Tbsp. prepared mustard
1 ½ cups Monterey Jack cheese shredded
1 ½ cups heavy cream
½ tsp. Old Bay seasoning
5 oz. American cheese
2 tsp. bottled hot sauce
2 tsp. prepared mustard
Parmesan cheese

Recipe continues...

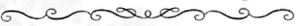

Notes:

First... spray a 9 inch pie plate with a non-stick spray.

Next... to the plate add shrimp, broccoli, celery, carrots, green onion and garlic. Mix so that all ingredients are distributed well.

Next... in bowl, add cream, milk, eggs, mustard, hot sauce, pepper, dill weed and Monterey Jack cheese. Pour over shrimp mixture. Top with Parmesan cheese.

Next... bake in 375 degree oven 45-60 minutes. Let stand 10 minutes before serving.

Next... add cream, American cheese, mustard, Old Bay and hot sauce. Simmer until mixture thickens. It should be smooth and glossy, coating the back of a spoon. It could take a few minutes to get there, but it will get thicker the longer it cooks.

Next... put a wedge of the egg bake on a plate and top with the Creole sauce and garnish with sweet paprika and dried parsley. Add some grapes or oranges if desired.

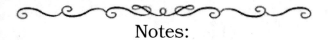

Notes:

Roadside Diner Cheeseburger Pie

Craving a cheeseburger? See if this will help you through your darkest hour! Who doesn't love a fabulous cheeseburger? And why shouldn't you have one!

9 inch pie plate
1 ½ cups ground beef, cooked and drained
1 cup diced roma tomatoes
½ cup chopped red or white onion
½ cup crumbled bacon
½ cup chopped pickle
1 cup cream
2 tsp. bottled hot sauce
½ cup milk
1 ½ c. shredded cheddar cheese
5 eggs
salt and pepper
1 Tbsp. prepared mustard

Recipe continues...

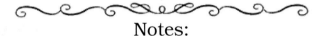

Notes:

First... spray pie plate with non-stick spray. Heat oven to 375 degrees.

Next... in pie plate, put beef, tomatoes, onion, bacon and pickle. Mix well to make sure it is all blended.

Next... in bowl, add cream, milk, eggs, mustard, hot sauce, cheese and salt and pepper. Beat well until thoroughly mixed. Pour over meat mixture. Top with more cheese and some Parmesan cheese if you desire.

Next... bake in oven for 45-60 minutes or until center is set. Cool for ten minutes before serving.

Next... place a lettuce leaf on a plate. Place a wedge of the cheeseburger pie on the plate. Top with a thin tomato slice, thin red or white onion slice and a dab of Mayo on top of it. Place a piece of diced tomato and a bacon bit in the middle of the Mayo. You're gonna love this one... I guarantee!

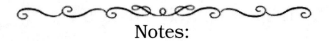

Notes:

Captain's Cove Seafood Salad

Ladies... this is perfect for a luncheon, but more than that it is perfect any time. Try this poolside... or at an elegant dinner party. It really is awesome!

2 lbs. cooked jumbo shrimp
1 lb. imitation lobster meat
2 cans crab meat, drained
2 cups Mayo (not Miracle Whip)
2 tsp. prepared Mustard
2 Tbsp. champagne vinegar or white wine
1 tsp. cracked pepper
5 Tbsp. fresh dill or two tsp. dried dill
1 pkg. dry Italian dressing mix
1 cup minced red onion
3 cups minced celery

First... remove tails from the shrimp. Shred lobster meat. Drain crab meat. Chop celery and onion.

Next... in separate bowl, whisk together the Mayo, mustard, wine or vinegar, Italian dressing mix, 1 tsp. salt, pepper and dill.

Next... combine the Mayo mixture with the seafood. Add the red onion and the celery. Check the seasonings. Cover and refrigerate for a few hours so that the spices can meld together.

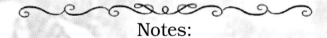

Notes:

TIP: A fun way to serve this salad is to buy those little dishes that look like half sea shells (you can get them in plastic or glass at the party stores) and pile the salad into the middle of the shell. Sprinkle with paprika and garnish with a lemon wedge. Add some dried parsley flakes. My friend Sadie likes to add chopped hard-boiled eggs to this salad... because she loves hard-boiled eggs!

TIP: To stop your hard cheese blocks from turning moldy in a plastic bag, wrap the cheese in a paper towel and then put it into the bag. It is the moisture that adheres to the cheese that turns it moldy!

Little Cindy Lou's Balsamic Honey Glazed Pork Medallions

If you have never tried a balsamic glaze before, I highly suggest that you try it. It's an explosion of flavor to your senses!

2 lb. pork tenderloin
½ cup good balsamic vinegar
3 Tbsp. honey
2 Tbsp. olive oil
1 Tbsp. chopped fresh rosemary (or 1 tsp. dried)
coarse salt and cracked pepper
green onions, chopped
1 tsp. minced garlic

recipe continues...

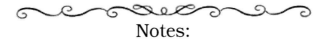

Notes:

First... add the vinegar, honey, olive oil, rosemary, salt, garlic and pepper. Whisk vigorously to emulsify. Adjust seasonings.

Next... slice tenderloin on the diagonal into one inch pieces. Heat a skillet with a little olive oil until hot. Sear medallions on each side and transfer to baking dish. (Preheat oven to 350). Pour some of the glaze over the medallions.

Next... roast 8-10 minutes (do not over cook) and transfer to a serving platter. Drizzle remainder of the glaze over the medallions and garnish with rosemary and green onions.

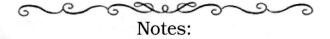

Notes:

TIP: You can add some Mandarin orange sections to your platter with the medallions. The flavor combination is really nice and it makes a wonderful presentation!

Annie Moss' Chicken Fantasy

Every bite of this chicken is as succulent as it can get! Make up extra and you will have it on hand for later in the week. You won't be sorry... this truly is wonderful!

8 frozen, boneless, skinless chicken breasts, thawed
1 cup Parmesan cheese
2 cups mushrooms, sliced
2 cups heavy cream
a little wine of choice, Marsala, Madeira, whatever you like
fresh rosemary, chopped or you can use dried
½ lb. bacon, diced but not cooked
coarse salt and cracked black pepper

First... sauté chicken, mushrooms and bacon in a 9x13 pan on top of the stove until browned but not completely done.

Next... remove from stove and add heavy cream, rosemary, wine, salt and pepper and top with Parmesan cheese.

Next... preheat oven to 350 degrees. When oven is ready, put chicken breasts in and finish baking for 30 minutes or so, depending on the size of the breasts. You do not want to over bake them because they will dry out.

Next... serve with a steamed or sautéed vegetable or fresh fruit. If you are doing the no carb thing... omit veggie and fruit.

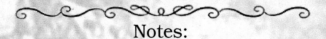

Notes:

TIP: When you use bottled spices, always pour a little of the spices into the palm of your hand and crush them with the thumb of your other hand. This will release the oils and freshen them up a bit. You can also roast seeds like coriander in a dry skillet and then grind them in a coffee grinder.

Rasta Mom's Island Lime Chicken Breasts in a Nest

Here is one for fun. It is as exotic as it is exquisite! Escape to a tropical island. Create a mood, that's what it's all about!

4-6 frozen, boneless, skinless chicken breasts, thawed
2 limes, juiced and zested
1 tsp. ground cumin
2 tsp. finely chopped cilantro
2 Tbsp. honey
3 Tbsp. extra virgin olive oil
coarse salt and cracked black pepper
lettuce and carrot, very finely shredded
    (about 1 cup per breast)

First... blend first five ingredients in bowl. Sprinkle chicken breasts with salt and pepper. Coat chicken breasts with dressing mix and marinate 20-30 minutes.

Next... finely shred the lettuce and carrots into bowl. Grate zest of one lime into bowl. Sprinkle with lime juice, a drizzle of honey, olive oil and salt and pepper. Give a good toss.

Next... grill the chicken breasts on an indoor or outdoor grill. (Can use regular skillet, but it tastes better on a grill) Grill about 6-7 minutes per side but do not over cook or they will dry out.

Next... cut chicken breasts on the diagonal in about half inch slices. Place about one cup of lettuce mixture in the middle of the plate and arrange sliced chicken breast in the middle of the mixture. Garnish with more chopped cilantro or dried parsley. Drizzle a little more olive oil on top of the chicken breast, a little more honey also, if you like. Yummy!

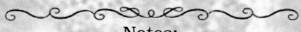

Notes:

Chu Chu's Chinese BBQ Pork Nests

These are as tasty as can be! Serve this at a party and they'll be gone before you turn around. We did! This is a proven hit! We hope you will like it.

1- (2 lb.) pork tenderloin
½ cup soy sauce
1 tsp. salt
½ cup Hoisin sauce
½-1 tsp. five spice powder
¼ cup oil
2 Tbsp. Cream Sherry
4-6 drops of red food coloring

First... mix all ingredients for marinade into bowl. Place tenderloin in zip lock baggie. Add the marinade in the zip lock baggie. Let the pork marinate overnight if possible. At least 4 hours.

Next... remove pork from marinade and place on rack in roaster pan, uncovered. Bake 350 degrees, 25-30 minutes, turning once or twice until done in the middle. Remove from pan and let it rest for 10 minutes to redistribute juices.

Recipe continues...

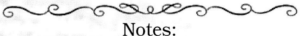

Notes:

Chu Chu's Chinese BBQ Pork Nests (Cont'd)

4 cups finely shredded lettuce
½ cup Hoisin sauce
½ cup finely shredded carrots
2 tsp. soy sauce
1 can water chestnuts, drained and chopped
2 Tbsp. oil
1 red bell pepper, seeded and diced
¼ tsp. five spice

First... shred the lettuce and carrots finely. Drain and chop the Water chestnuts and add them to the lettuce and carrots.

Next... mix the Hoisin sauce, soy sauce, oil and five spice and whisk vigorously to emulsify.

Next... to serve, place once cup of the lettuce mixture onto a plate and drizzle with the Hoisin dressing. Slice the tenderloin on the diagonal into ½ inch slices and place several neatly over the bed of lettuce. Drizzle a little more Hoisin dressing over the meat. If desired, you can add a few Mandarin orange slices on the plate next to the meat. This is a very nice flavor combination.

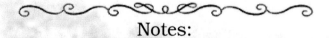

Notes:

Yes! Those Mandarin oranges do get a work out in this book! Why? Because frankly.... They are so appealing with everything. They are just a natural flavor enhancer and balancer. Try different fruits. We do, we just happen to prefer the oranges.

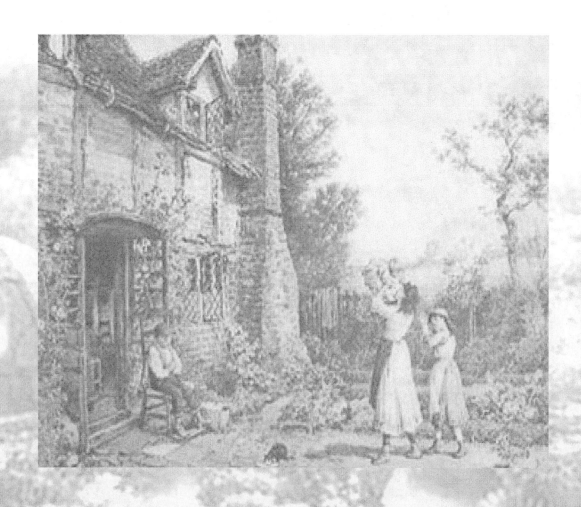

Shrimp Shack Seafood Platter with Sassy Sally's Lip Smackin' Tartar Sauce

1-2 sea bass or other nice white fillet
12-16 jumbo sea scallops
12-16 jumbo shrimp
sauce for seafood

6 Tbsp. melted butter
2 Tbsp. white wine
½ dill weed
½ minced garlic
2 lemons (cut into 4 wedges each)
cellophane noodles, prepared according to package
1 small can Mandarin oranges, drained

First... cut fish into 6-8 pieces each and arrange on foiled and oiled jelly roll pan. Arrange scallops and shrimp around fish. Drizzle with sauce below and bake 400 degrees until everything is white and fish is flakey. Do not over bake. Approximate baking time: 10 minutes.

Next... for the sauce... combine all ingredients except lemon wedges, cellophane noodles and oranges. Drizzle over fish and seafood while baking.

Next... to prepare platter: line a platter with a dark leaf lettuce.

Next... add a layer of prepared cellophane noodles, leaving a hole in the middle for the tartar sauce bowl. Arrange seafood on platter. Sprinkle with paprika. Garnish with lemon wedges and Mandarin oranges.

Now... dip seafood into Sassy Sally's lip smackin' tartar sauce and enjoy!

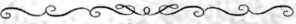

Notes:
Hands down... this is so awesome... I'm in heaven with this one!

Sassy Sally's Lip Smackin' Tartar Sauce

2 cups Mayo (not Miracle Whip)
½ to 1 tsp. Old Bay seasoning
1 ½ Tbsp. lemon juice
1-2 tsp. hot sauce
¼ cup of finely minced red bell pepper
½ cup minced onion
1 tsp. prepared mustard
¼ cup pickle relish
1/3 cup buttermilk
coarse salt

First... combine all ingredients. Store in covered container in ice box several hours or overnight. The longer it sits the better the flavors will marry.

If you want to try something different, substitute one cup of diced and seeded roma tomatoes for the one cup of bell peppers in this recipe. It is every bit as good if not better.

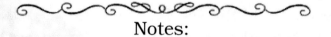

Notes:

Do something nice for yourself. If you want to feel refreshed in the morning after waking up, put a few drops of eucalyptus or peppermint oil on a tissue. Stand outside the back door in the fresh air... Put the tissue up to your nose, breath in, exhale. Fill you lungs with fresh outside air. How exhilarating! Repeat as desired.

Remember... sometimes the biggest let downs in life are our own expectations!

Captain Earl's Cranberry Orange Stuffed Chicken Breast

If cranberries are not your thing, don't let that stop you from trying this one! This is a five star dish and certainly a signature entrée around here! It's a layering of flavors that will explode with every mouth-watering bite you take.

6-8 Boneless, skinless chicken breasts
5 oz. Swiss Almond cheese spread
½ cup ricotta cheese
1 egg
½ tsp. allspice
2 tsp. minced garlic
1 cup fresh chopped spinach
½ cup chopped Mandarin orange sections
½ cup dried cranberries

Sauce:

1 ½ cups heavy cream
½ cup Marsala or Sherry
½ cup orange juice
½ cup dried cranberries
salt and pepper
allspice to taste

Cont'd.....

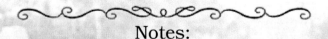

Notes:

First... take a sharp knife and slice through the thickest end of the chicken breast, going in as far as possible to make a pocket.

Next... mix all the stuffing ingredients in a bowl. Spoon as much stuffing into each pocket as you can get. I use an ice cream scooper. Place chicken breasts in roasting pan sprayed with non-stick spray.

Next... make the sauce by placing all the sauce ingredients in a sauce pan and simmering at low heat, until sauce thickens slightly. It will become darker in color and it should coat the back of a spoon. It should look smooth and glossy. It could take a few minutes, but the longer you simmer it, the thicker it will become.

Next... pour the sauce over the chicken breasts and bake in 350 degree oven for around 30 minutes or until done. Do not over cook because the chicken breasts will become dry. Add more sauce if needed.

Next... serve on a plate and garnish with more oranges, cranberries and if desired, dried parsley.

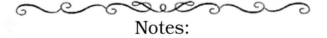

Notes:

Sunny Creek's Walleye Supreme

This is what you call jazzed up fish! You can use any nice white fish fillet. This is so good. The fillets should be at least ¾ inch thick to start off with.

      1 lb. Walleye or any other nice white fish fillet
      8 oz. grated cheddar cheese
      8 oz. sour cream
      ½ cup heavy cream
      1 tsp. dried tarragon
      1 medium onion, diced

First... heat oven to 350 degrees.

Next... place fish in shallow bake dish. Sprinkle diced onion and cheese over top of fish.

Next... mix all other ingredients and spoon over the fish.

Next... bake 30 minutes, checking to make sure that you do not over bake the fish, if you do it will become rubbery. Sprinkle with lemon juice if desired.

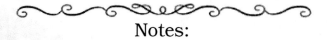

Notes:

TIP: Sprinkle with lemon juice before serving. Garnish with a little dried parsley or tarragon if you wish.

Are we having fun yet? I'm having fun just being able to share these recipes with you.

Brother Gary's Veal Marsala Wala Bing Bang

You can really use whatever meat you desire in this dish. Chicken works well too. We all know this dish is out of this world, and we certainly don't want just the ordinary now do we?   Why do we have to go to a restaurant to get it? Make it at home!

1 ½ lbs. veal cutlets for Scaloppini, (thinned out)
½ cup flour
5 Tbsp. butter
¼ cup olive oil
1 large shallot, minced
2 lbs. Cremini (baby portabella) mushrooms
1 cup Marsala wine
½ cup beef stock (canned is preferable over cubes)

Recipe continues...

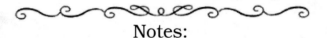

Notes:

First... season veal with salt and pepper. Dredge meat in flour.

Next... preheat large skillet over medium high heat. For each batch of meat, use 1 Tbsp. butter and 1 Tbsp. olive oil in pan. (it will take more than one batch to sauté the meat).

Next... sauté cutlets in a single layer and cook for 2 minutes each side. Place on warm serving platter. Cook the next batch and so on, adding to the warm serving platter.

Next... after the meat is sautéed, add the rest of the ingredients to pan and simmer for a few minutes. Cook down to evaporate some of the liquid. Return the meat to the skillet, and continue cooking a couple of minutes. Remove from heat and transfer to a serving platter. Garnish with dried parsley.

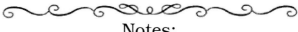

Notes:

This dish is served without egg noodles. However, if you miss the noodles and need a little something extra, a little side of cottage cheese or a clump of green grapes works well. If you are not worried about a few carbs, go ahead and have the noodles.

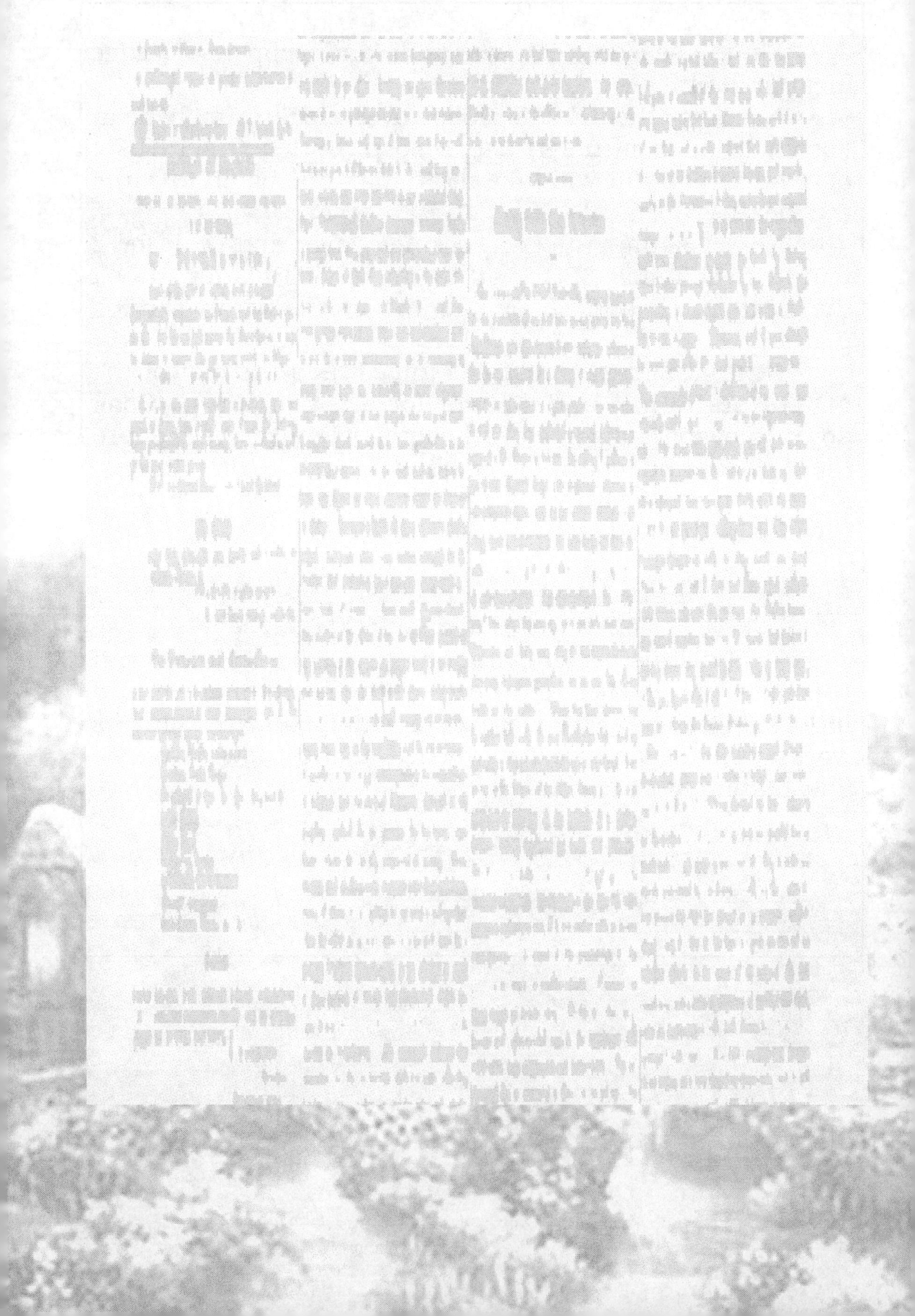

Rasta Mom and Jimmy Jam's Island Shrimp

Nothing like a sunset in Negril and a platter of Island Shrimp to top it all off! This is certainly an absolute addiction! Sail away!

1 cup coconut
2 tsp. chopped cilantro
½ cup orange juice
½ cup lime juice
½ tsp. jerk seasoning
¼ cup honey
2 or more lbs. jumbo shrimp (deveined but shell on)
¼ cup oil
1 tsp. minced garlic

First... mix marinade in bowl. Transfer to a zip lock baggie. Place shrimp in baggie for about 45 minutes to marinate. After 45 minutes, drain shrimp and discard marinade.

Next... in a skillet, heat 2 tsp. oil until hot but not smoking. Throw in a few shrimp and sauté until pink. Do not over cook. These will only take a couple of minutes. The shell on helps to protect the shrimp from over cooking. Remove from pan to serving platter and re-load the skillet with more shrimp. Continue process until all shrimp are sautéed and are on the serving platter. Now remove shells and garnish with lime wedges.

Next... once platter is loaded with shrimp, sprinkle with toasted coconut. Toast coconut by taking a cup of coconut and spreading out on a jelly roll pan and broiling until slightly browned. This will take only a couple of seconds under the broiler.

Next... serve with jerk marmalade. Add a bowl of this marmalade to the center of the platter.

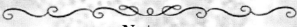

Notes:

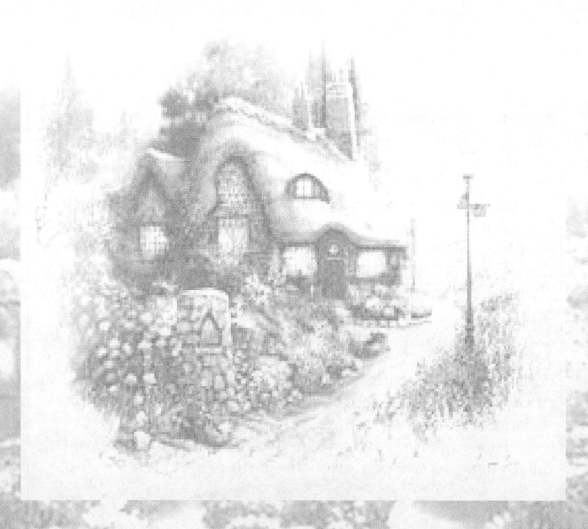

Jerk Marmalade

1 cup marmalade, 1 Tbsp. lime juice and zest from on lime, ½ tsp. jerk seasoning and toasted coconut to taste. Mix well and transfer to pretty bowl. This is the greatest dip for this shrimp... OK! I have to have the marmalade! I just have to. Caution!!! This dip has carbs in it. Maybe you will want to save up for this one! That's what we do! That's life! Eat sparingly... yeah, right! Let's be real... we have to live. This is absolutely awesome! This is spoken like a true carb-junkie. See what I mean? We're all human! Do save up! Eat sparingly. Don't go crazy!...really! I mean that!

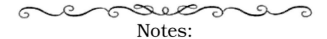

Notes:

Do you want to change a mood? Have you ever thought of having a theme dinner just for fun? They are a blast! Not only are they a blast to plan them, they are a blast to attend.

Have a Mexican fiesta. Decorate your room, table, chairs, candles and tablecloths. Have a Mexican pot luck or buffet. Dress for the occasion.

Try a Hawaiian luau, a Tex Mex meal, a candle light dinner for two. Have some fun with it. If you have a patio, light it up with lights and candles. Hang up some fabric of the same theme. Dress up the table.

Do some color themes... all red... all black... do a black tie!

How about a "Hot Arabian Night Dinner?" A jungle theme? Do it yourself or get your guests involved, right down to the invitations and the table settings.

How about a 30's, 40's or 50's dinner night? The sky is the limit. You know you need a change of pace once and a while. You may not think this is for you, but don't say this until you have tried it! It really is a blast and it gives people something to do, out of the ordinary, and that's what we need sometimes... out of the ordinary!

A lot of these props and dishes etc. can be found in the thrift stores every where for pennies on the dollar. Try the garage sales, they are good places also. Use your imagination. Go crazy, have some fun. Save the accessories for future use or give them to someone else and encourage them to use them. Have a very romantic Valentines Day party. Make it a dress up affair. Play romantic music to dance to. Have a romantic dinner and invite some friends... make it a couples thing. People really will have fun!

Crab Shack Jack's Jumbo Scallops with an Awesome Woozie Citrus Sauce

1-2 lbs. fresh jumbo scallops
2 tsp. minced garlic
¼ cup Tequila
2 tsp. lime zest
½ cup lime juice
3 Tbsp. fresh mint, chopped
2 Tbsp. honey
salt and pepper to taste
½ cup olive oil

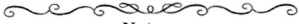

Notes:

You can use some cilantro if you like. Remember, cilantro has a strong flavor, so use it to your taste.

Put scallops in a large zip lock baggie. In bowl, mix the rest of the ingredients. Pour into zip lock baggie over scallops. Marinate 30-60 minutes.

Next... remove scallops from the marinade. Discard left over marinade.

Next... drizzle olive oil into skillet and heat well. Sear the scallops so that they are a little caramelized... done only to center. Do not over cook scallops or they will turn rubbery.

Next... remove scallops to serving platter lined with banana leaves if you can find them, or be creative and come up with your own idea for presentation.

Next... in same skillet, add a little more oil and reheat pan. Add lime zest and juice of one lime. Add 1 tsp. minced garlic, 1 oz. Tequila, 1 tsp. chopped mint and 1 Tbsp. honey. Sauté 1-2 minutes. Remove from heat and add 5 Tbsp. cold butter and whisk to incorporate. Drizzle onto scallops.

Next... add some lemon and lime wedges to the platter. And add some Mandarin orange sections if you wish for color. The flavor combination between the oranges and scallops is wonderful. Garnish with parsley, mint or cilantro.

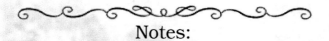

Notes:

Unbelievable Turkey Burgers from the Bog

These burgers are so incredible... that even if you don't care for turkey, you might change your mind. These burgers rock!

   2 lbs. fresh ground turkey, not frozen
   1 small apple, peeled and grated
   1 small onion, minced
   1 stalk celery, finely
   1 tsp. poultry seasoning
   ¼ cup whole cranberry sauce
   coarse salt and cracked black pepper

First... combine all the above ingredients and mix well. Shape into large patties. If you are really hungry... make them into a third pound or half pound burger.

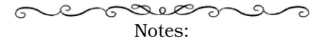

Notes:

Bog Sauce (Cont'd)

½ cup Mayo (not Miracle Whip)
2 Tbsp. whole cranberry sauce
salt and pepper to taste

Next... mix the ingredients for the sauce well and let sit for a few minutes.

Next... fry the turkey burgers in skillet for about 6-8 minutes each side or until done in the middle. Do not over cook.

Next... transfer burgers to serving dish and add sauce to the top of the burger. Garnish with a clump or grapes or some orange sections or try a couple of apple slices.

If you are looking for a burger with a little different taste... this is it! This is certainly number one on the Cottage House menu.

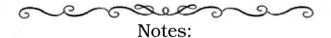

Notes:

Are you a pasta lover? Actually, a Fettuccine Alfredo lover? If you are craving your Alfredo, maybe we can help.

Try this recipe. It was passed on to me. I know quite a few people who really like this substitute for the pasta noodles.

Buy some Japanese egg plant, or regular egg plant would work. Peel and julienne the egg plant meat into thin strips about the size of fettuccine noodles. They will shrink down when you sauté them. Keep that in mind and make more than you think you will need. Put them in a colander and sprinkle liberally with salt (this will extract the water from the strips). Let them sit in the colander for about 30 minutes. Squeeze the remaining water from the strips by placing them between a paper towel and pressing the liquid out. Sauté in butter but do not over cook them because they will turn mushy. Try them with Alfredo or spaghetti sauce. Spaghetti sauce does contain some carbs, so watch the count.

Creamy Alfredo Sauce

1 stick butter, sliced
1 (8oz.) package cream cheese
¾ fresh Parmesan cheese, grated
2 cups heavy cream
garlic salt and white pepper to taste

In sauce pan, melt butter over medium heat. Add cream cheese and Parmesan. Whisk until smooth. Add garlic and pepper and stir until everything is blended together.

This also makes a great sauce for vegetables or you can use it for chicken with mushrooms.

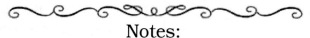

Notes:

The best things in life are free. Hugs, smiles, compassion, devotion, compliments, an act of kindness... and since they are free... what stops us from giving more of it away?

Beachcomber Bob's Seafood Newburg

6 Tbsp. butter, divided in half
white pepper to taste
2 small bay leaves
cayenne pepper to taste
2 medium shallots, minced
½ lb. large shrimp, peeled
3 Tbsp. flour or arrowroot
½ lb. scallops
¼ tsp. paprika
½ lb. crabmeat
1½ tsp. chicken base
½ cup Cream Sherry
2 cups heavy cream
1 tsp. lemon zest

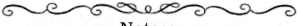

Notes:

This should be against the law it is so good! This is what I mean... how can you feel like you are giving up anything good to eat when you have all these goodies? Is this terrific?

First... melt 3 Tbsp. butter in large saucepan. Add bay leaves and shallots and sauté two minutes until tender and fragrant. Stir in flour or arrowroot and enough paprika to give the roux a nice rich red color. Cook, stirring about 3 minutes, until it thickens. Slowly add heavy cream, lemon zest and chicken base and stir until sauce thickens. Season with peppers. Keep cream sauce warm.

Next... in a skillet, melt the other 3 Tbsp. butter over medium high heat. Add seafood and sauté about 2 minutes or just until cooked through. Do not over cook, it will turn rubbery.

Next... Transfer seafood to cream sauce with slotted spoon. Add Sherry to skillet and using wooden spoon, losen and scrape any of the little bits off the bottom of the pan. Stir Sherry into cream sauce. Take out bay leaves and serve in an elegant dish. Garnish with fresh or dried parsley and lemon wedges. You can purchase little sea shell dishes in plastic or glass at the party stores... this is a fun way to present your dish.

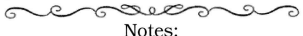

Notes:

TIP: The color of the sauce should be about the color of tomato soup with the milk added to it. Pinkish red.

I'm sure that by now you have figured out that some recipes are hard to do without bread crumbs.

We have found a solution that work's really well. The solution is pork rinds in the bag. Yes! That's right! The kind the guys like to eat all the time. Maybe some of you gals like them, but for the most part, I bet you are going to turn your nose up at this. Before you do that, read on!

The pork rind has been absolutely under-rated! There are no carbohydrates and they are guilt free. They are crunchy and can be disguised in flavor much the same way tofu picks up the flavor of the dish you are using it in. Here are some of the things that we have discovered we can use them for, and they are great! Give them a chance.

These guys can replace those potato chips and nacho chips at parties and you can still have something to dip, with no Carbs, and they are stronger, less breakable in dip!

As a topping for a green bean casserole... crunch some up, add a little melted butter, some garlic salt, and dehydrated onion flakes and you have the equivalent of those french fried onion rings in the can. Use them to top of any vegetable dish.

Crunch them up or buzz them in the food processor and use instead of flour to make a quick pie crust with melted butter and Splenda and pat into a pie pan. Use them for your quiches if you want the crunch of a topping.

For snacks toss them with melted butter and any herb or cheese topping. Try Cajun, southwest, dill, garlic salt... use your imagination.

Use them as croutons in a salad or French onion soup.

As a sweet snack... crunch up a bunch of pork rinds, toss with melted butter, cinnamon and Splenda and you have a sweet crunchy snack.

Grind them fine and use them in place of bread crumbs in a meat loaf recipe.

Break them up in chunks, toss them in butter and coat them with dry ranch dressing mix... they are good!

Dip them in melted, sugar free chocolate, or if you are not worried about a couple of carbs, use semi-sweet... the real deal.

Ground them up and use them as breading for a turkey patty, hamburger patty to make chicken fried steak, chicken breast or any other meat. Season them with herbs and spices before dipping meat into them. Use an egg wash before you dip, then just fry.

MaMa Chula's Jerk Chicken Breasts with Crazy Cucumber Dipping Sauce

Jerk Marinade:

1 onion, finely chopped
½ tsp cinnamon
½ cup finely chopped scallions
1 tsp. cracked pepper
½ tsp. poultry seasoning
3 Tbsp. soy sauce
1 tsp. salt
1 Tbsp. cooking oil
3 tsp, Splenda
1 Tbsp. cider vinegar
2 lbs. boneless, skinless chicken Breasts
½ tsp. allspice

First... mix all these ingredients plus chicken and put in a covered container.   Refrigerate until ready to use. May add some fresh chopped cilantro as well.

Next... grill chicken breasts on the inside or outside grill. You can use a skillet also, but they taste better if you grill them.

Next... cut chicken breasts on the diagonal into strips about ½ inch to 1 inch wide. Place on platter with bowl of "Crazy Cucumber" dipping sauce (from this book) in the middle. Add a few grape or cherry tomatoes to the platter for color and you can dip them also. Add lime wedges to the platter for squeezing onto the chicken breasts.

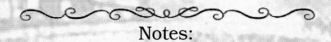

Notes:

Blue Lagoon's Surf and Turf

2 nice approximately 8 oz. Filet Mignon
½ lb. jumbo shrimp, cooked, de-veined and
    de-shelled

Béarnaise sauce:

2 shallots, finely minced
½ cup white wine
4 ½ tsp. chopped fresh tarragon or 1 tsp. dried
½ cup champagne vinegar
Freshly ground black pepper
4 large egg yolks
2 sticks butter, cut into small pieces
1½ tsp. chopped fresh chervil
Salt

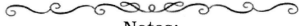

Notes:
Serve this by candle light and you have the perfect special occasion dinner. Valentine's Day, Anniversary, Birthday... make it special! It doesn't get much better than this!

First... salt and pepper both sides of the filet mignon.

Next... make the Béarnaise sauce. Combine shallots, wine, vinegar, 1 Tbsp. tarragon (or the 1 tsp. dried), and two pinches of pepper in a small pot set over medium heat, and reduce to about two tablespoons. Set aside to cool.

Next... beat the egg yolks with 2 Tbsp. of water over low heat for about 2-3 minutes or until they become thick and foamy. Add the butter, about a Tbsp. at a time, whisking until the mixture thickens and increases in volume.

Next... add the shallot mixture, chervil, and the remaining tarragon. Season with salt and pepper and stir to combine. This will make one cup.

Next... heat an indoor grill or skillet until very hot but not smoking. Add oil. Place filets on the grill and cook for 3 minutes per side for medium rare. Remove from grill and transfer to dinner plate. Let set ten minutes to re-distribute the juices. Sauté shrimp quickly in butter. Do not over cook.

Next... add the shrimp to the Béarnaise sauce and heat just until warmed up. Divide the sauce and shrimp between the two plates. Pour the sauce over the Filet Mignon. Garnish the plate with more tarragon or parsley, whatever you choose. Garnish with a clump of green or red grapes.

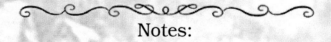

Notes:

Here is a romantic little low carb desert that you can serve with the Blue Lagoon's Surf and Turf to top it off in grand style!

Little Love Nests

2 martini glasses or similar glasses
1 no-bake cheese cake, sugar free if possible
½ cup heavy cream
1 Tbsp. butter
2 oz. unsweetened baking chocolate 60gr. thick
1 tsp. vanilla
1/3 cup Splenda
4 or more large strawberries

First... prepare cheese cake according to directions on the box. Pour cheese cake into each glass, ¾ of the way full. Let set.

Next... place cream, chocolate and butter in a small sauce pan. Heat almost to boiling. Whisk chocolate into the cream.

Next... remove from heat, stir in vanilla and Splenda, mix well. Let cool for about 10 minutes. Spoon a layer of chocolate over the top of the cheese cake. Top with two strawberries each... flat side down. Put them together in the middle of the glass. Press in somewhat to make sure they become secure. Chill until ready to enjoy! How romantic!

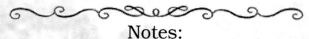

Notes:

TIP: *Something else you can do to the cheese cake to make it different would be to take a couple of drops of red food coloring and just swirl it through the cheese cake. Try different flavorings too.*

Tequila Lime Dressing

½ cup white Tequila
½ tsp. coarse salt
2 Tbsp. fresh lime juice
¼ tsp. cracked black pepper
2 Tbsp. minced shallots
¼ cup heavy cream
1 tsp. minced garlic
1 stick butter, cut up at room temp
1 Tbsp. fresh chopped cilantro
1-2 Tbsp. honey

First... combine the Tequila, lime juice, honey, shallots, garlic, cilantro, salt, and pepper in a sauce pan over high heat and bring to a boil. Reduce liquid by half. Stir in the cream and simmer for 3 minutes. Add the butter and remove from heat. Continue whisking until the butter is incorporated. Cool slightly and drizzle over salads. Use this dressing with "Shrimp Salad on Glass".

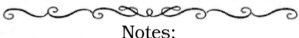

Notes:

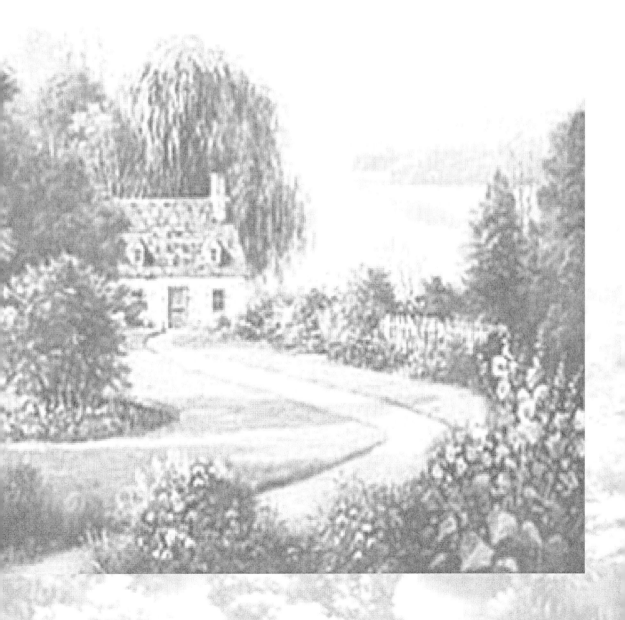

Cappie's Shrimp Salad on Glass

You can surely impress your Mother-In-Law with this one! So refreshing, especially on those hot summer days.

2 lb. medium shrimp, cooked, de-veined and tails off
1/3 cup lime juice
1/3 cup lemon juice
2 tsp. Splenda
1 tsp. fresh mint, chopped
3 roma tomatoes, diced small

1 hand full cilantro, stemmed, chopped fine
2 avocados

1 cucumber, peeled, seeded, diced small
1 red onion, diced small

First: Place shrimp in gallon sized zip lock baggie. In bowl add the lemon, lime and orange juice. Add Splenda and fresh mint. Add marinade to shrimp. close tightly and marinate 4-6 hours.

Next: In bowl, put tomatoes, cilantro, cucumber and red onion. Let sit at room temperature 20 min. Do not peel the avocado until you remove the shrimp from marinade, then peel, pit and dice.

Next: Remove shrimp from marinade with slotted spoon and add to other ingredients. Now you can add the peeled, pitted and diced avocado. Put salad mix in chilled martini glasses and top with Tequila Lime Dressing. (Recipe from book). Garnish with mint or cilantro.

Freaky Freddie's Fish Dish

2-4 white fish fillets, any white fish will do
4-6 Tbsp. butter
dill weed
coarse salt and cracked pepper
lemon pepper seasoning

Place fish fillets in a shallow baking dish. Pour melted butter over the fish and season with seasoning. Bake 375 degrees for approximately 10-15 minutes depending on size of the fillets. Make sure fish will flake easily but do not over bake.

Next... make salsa:

½ cup drained Mandarin orange slices, chopped
¼ cup red onion, diced
½ cup roma tomatoes, seeded and diced
¼ cup green onion, chopped
1 lime, use juice and zest
3 Tbsp. Italian dressing
chopped cilantro to taste

Mix all ingredients for salsa and either chill, to let the flavors meld together, or if necessary you can use it right away.

Next... place baked fish fillets on serving platter and spoon salsa over the fillets. Garnish with cilantro or parsley. If you can get banana leaves, it always looks nice to place a couple of the leaves on the plate before you put down the fish and salsa. It's great for parties.

Notes:

DESSERTS
And now...some sweet treats from The Cottage House
After all...what is a meal without dessert?

Notes:

Cabot Cove's Black Forest Cheese Cake

Cheese Cake and Ganache mixture:

4- (8 oz.) pkgs. cream cheese, softened
1 cup cream
3 eggs
2 Tbsp. butter
¾ cup Splenda
4 oz. unsweetened
½ tsp. almond extract
baking chocolate
½ cup heavy cream
1 tsp. vanilla
2/3 cup Splenda

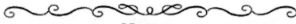

Notes:
Ganache glazed cheese cake? You won't even believe how decadent this little number is... and you can have it! Someone wake me up!

First... set oven to 325 degrees.

Next... beat cream cheese in bowl until smooth. Add eggs, beating well after each addition. Add sugar and almond extract. Beat until smooth. Add ½ cup heavy cream and blend well.

Next... pour into a well sprayed 9 or 10 inch spring form pan. Bake 1 hour and 15 minutes or until middle is set. Middle should still be a little loose. I like to lay a piece of foil over the top of the cheese cake to stop the top from browning while baking. Don't fasten it down, just lay it over top.

Next... cool on wire rack one hour and then refrigerate overnight. Refrigerating overnight is critical because you will not achieve the texture if you don't.

Next... place cream, chocolate and butter in small pan. Heat until almost boiling. Whisk to combine chocolate with cream. Remove from heat. Stir in vanilla and Splenda making sure to mix well. Cool for ten minutes.

Next... remove cheese cake from spring form pan ring. Place a wire rack on top of a jelly roll pan and place the cheese cake on top of it.

Next... whisk chocolate until it starts to thicken. Pour over the cheese cake, making sure to cover the whole thing. Cover twice if necessary and ganache permitting. Top with a couple of strawberries in the center of the cake. Chill and enjoy!

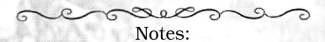

Notes:

TIP: If you would like to make a strawberry sauce to go over the cheesecake pieces after you have cut them, pick tops off of strawberries, slice and add enough Splenda to cover them. Let them sit until the strawberries make their own sauce. Spoon over the cheese cake.

Little Love Nests

        martini or margarita glasses
        1 no-bake cheese cake (sugar free if possible)
        1 cup cream
        2 Tbsp. butter
        4 oz. unsweetened baking chocolate, 60gr. thick
        1 tsp. vanilla
        2/3 cup Splenda
        4 or more large strawberries

First... prepare cheese cake according to directions on the box. Pour cheese cake into each glass ¾ of the way full. Let sit.

Next... place cream, chocolate and butter in a small sauce pan. Heat almost to boiling. Whisk chocolate into the cream. Remove from heat, stir in vanilla and Splenda, and mix well. Let cool for 10 minutes. Spoon a layer of chocolate over the top of the cheese cake. Top with two strawberries each, flat side down. Put them together in the middle of the glass. Press down some what to make sure they become secure. Chill until ready to enjoy! How romantic!

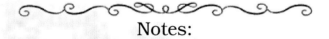

Notes:

TIP: Something else you can do to the cheese cake to make it different would be to take a couple of drops of red food coloring and just swirl it through the cheese cake mix. Try different extracts in the cheese cake mix, like strawberry, amaretto, peppermint, lemon, almond... you get the idea. Here is another suggestion, add a couple of drops of orange food coloring to the mix. Add some orange extract, a few chopped Mandarin orange pieces and top with the ganache and a Mandarin orange section on top of the chocolate.

Another suggestion would be to add a couple drops of green food coloring or a drop or two of peppermint extract. Top with the chocolate ganache and garnish with a mint leave and an Andes Cream de Menthe square. Just push it in the top of the chocolate so that it is sticking out of the chocolate about ¾ of the way. You can use any kind of chocolate covered mint. If you don't want to eat it, give it away as an angel wish to someone.

Another suggestion: Add melted unsweetened chocolate to the mix to make it chocolate cheese cake. Top with ganache, poke a mint square into the top and call it "death by chocolate". Something different all the time.

Tip: If you can not find a no-bake cheese cake that is sugar-free, use the regular and count the carbs in the cheese cake according to the box. If you would like this dessert but you have to have it sugar free, here is a similar idea. I have made the regular black forest cheese cake (sugar-free) without the chocolate ganache topping. When the cheese cake has been chilled over night, I use an ice cream scooper and scoop balls out of the cheese cake and put them in chilled martini or margarita glasses. 3 good size scoops and add a topping. Garnish with some of the suggestions mentioned earlier. When you get to know how to make this cheese cake with ease, you will be able to add extracts, flavorings and food colorings to the cheese cake base and just bake according to directions.

Crazy Jan's Heavenly Coconut Macaroons

2 cups of shredded coconut
14 packets of Splenda
4 egg whites
1 cup heavy cream
½ to 1 tsp. almond extract

First... mix cream with sweetener and extract. Add coconut and mix well. Let stand for one hour. If mix feels too dry after this time, add a little more cream.

Next... preheat oven to 350 degrees.

Next... beat egg whites until stiff peaks form. Fold into Coconut. Using a small ice cream scooper or teaspoon, drop a small ball of mixture on a well greased cookie sheet. If you are fortunate enough to have a couple of Silpats, they work great!

Next... Scoop out approximately 32 cookies. Bake until slightly browned, 12-15 minutes. If tops are not browned by this time, you can place them under the broiler for a few seconds, but watch carefully. Cool completely before serving.

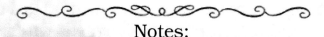

Notes:

TIP: here again, you can experiment with colorings and extracts. Use your imagination. We make pastels. Pink, yellow, blue and lavender for Easter. We take a pretty spring platter, line it with some Easter grass and add the cookies. It makes a lovely Easter dish for the table. Wrap them in little cellophanes and add them to the Easter baskets.

Another suggestion: Drizzle them with chocolate (sweetened with Splenda) or coat half or the entire cookie. Yum!

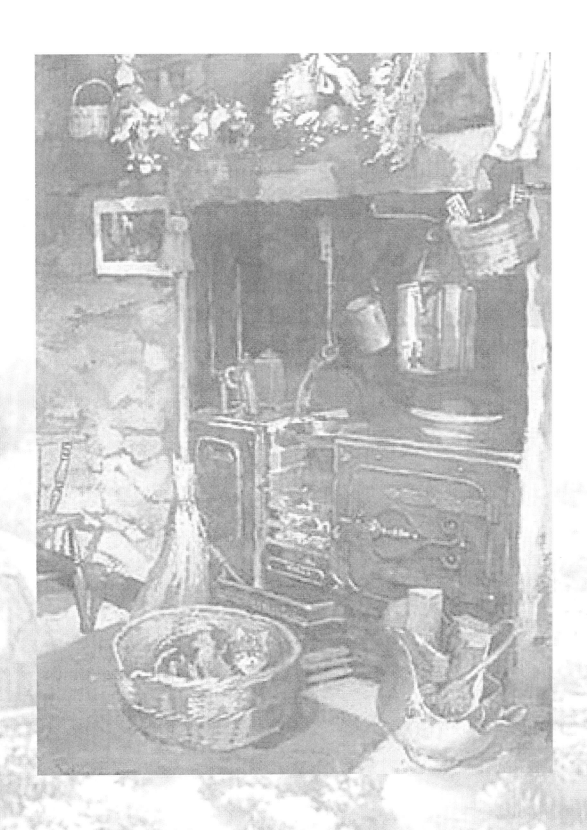

PaPa Mike's Sugar Free Fudge Land Express

Bringing you the fudge that you can actually eat a Christmas time, because Christmas just isn't Christmas without fudge, nor is any day a day without fudge... to the true chocolate lover. This fudge... 1 carb per piece, normal size.

½ cup butter
4 oz. unsweetened chocolate
2 cups Splenda
2 tsp. vanilla
1 lb. cream cheese, room temperature
macadamia nuts, cashews or pecans

First... melt butter over low heat. Add chocolate and stir until melted. Remove from heat and stir in sweetener and vanilla.

Next... combine chocolate mixture with cream cheese and beat until smooth. Stir in nuts if used and spread into a 9x13 pan greased pan.

Next... refrigerate until firm and keep in the refrigerator.

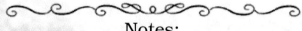

Notes:

TIP: you can add all kinds of extracts to the original recipe. Raspberry, mint, espresso, orange, peppermint. Have some fun with it. Pa Pa Mike likes to use rum flavoring, Miss Tina likes the strawberry extract.

Too Good To Be True... Tiramisu

You will actually dazzle the daylights out of your family and friends. This no carb, low carb thing just gets better all the time! About the only carbs in here come from the vanilla wafers. We picked the lowest carb wafers we could find.

1 lb. Mascarpone cheese
5 egg yolks
1/3 cup Splenda
1 tsp. almond extract
½ cup espresso coffee or very strong coffee
30 vanilla wafers, (Keebler is the least carbs)
2 tsp. cocoa powder
2 tsp. orange zest
heavy whipping cream and Splenda for topping

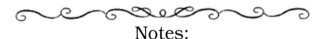

Notes:

First... brew the espresso or very strong coffee. Pour into container and refrigerate to chill.

Next... whisk together the Mascarpone, egg yolks, Splenda and almond extract until smooth. Set aside.

Next... bring out a pretty, clear glass dish or desert dish and line it with the vanilla wafers.

Next... quickly dip each wafer into the espresso and place into the dish to form a single layer. Be very careful not to get the wafers too wet or they will fall apart. Just dip them quickly!

Next... spoon the cheese mixture over the wafers and smooth out with the back of the spoon.

Next... take as much whipping cream as you think you might need and add a tsp. or two of Splenda and beat until stiff peaks form.

Next... spread a layer of whipped cream over the top of the Tiramisu and garnish with cocoa powder and orange zest. You can also garnish with shaved unsweetened chocolate curls. Refrigerate a good couple of hours so that it can set up. As if that isn't good enough... drizzle on some sugar-free chocolate sauce and garnish with a mint leave or two.

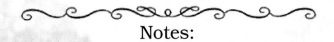

Notes:

Uncle Nunzio's Italian Strawberry Gelato

½ lb. fresh strawberries
6 oz. Splenda
2 oz. of cold heavy cream

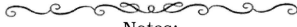

Notes:

If you have never tried Gelato before... you are in for a treat! The Italians' were way ahead of the game when it came to making ice cream. Gelato shops are every where in Italy. Gelato is smoother, creamier and fresher than any ice cream I know of here... and comes in tons of rich fresh fruity flavors as well as the custards. Great as a summer time treat, and great for an anytime treat. We think that once you try this, ice cream will take a back seat!

First... pull off the leaves and stems from the strawberries and cut the berries in half, unless they are very small. Wash them in cold water.

Next... put the strawberries with all of the sugar in the bowl of a food processor, process for a few moments, then add 7 oz. water and continue to process until liquefied.

Next... whip the cream until it thickens slightly, to the consistency of buttermilk. Put the cream and the pureed strawberries in a bowl and mix thoroughly. Chill until very cold.

Next... if you have an ice cream maker, pour the mixture, making sure it is very cold, into the container of your ice cream maker and freeze according to the manufacturer's instructions. When done, the Gelato is ready to eat, but if you want to serve it later, or prefer it when it is more compact, transfer it to a container that closes tightly and place in the freezer. If you are going to leave it in the freezer overnight or longer, let the Gelato soften a little by putting it in the refrigerator for 30 minutes before serving.

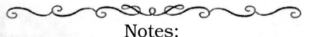

Notes:

No ice cream maker? If you do not have an ice cream maker, pour the cold mixture into a freezer container, close the lid tightly and place in the freezer until set... about 3 hours. Remove from the container and chop roughly into 3 pieces. Place in the bowl of a food processor and process until smooth (or use a fork). Return to the freezer and freeze again until firm. Repeat the freezing and chopping process 2 or 3 more times until a smooth consistency is reached. Serving suggestion: Spoon into martini or margarita glasses. Drizzle with sugar-free chocolate sauce and garnish with a fresh strawberry and mint leave.

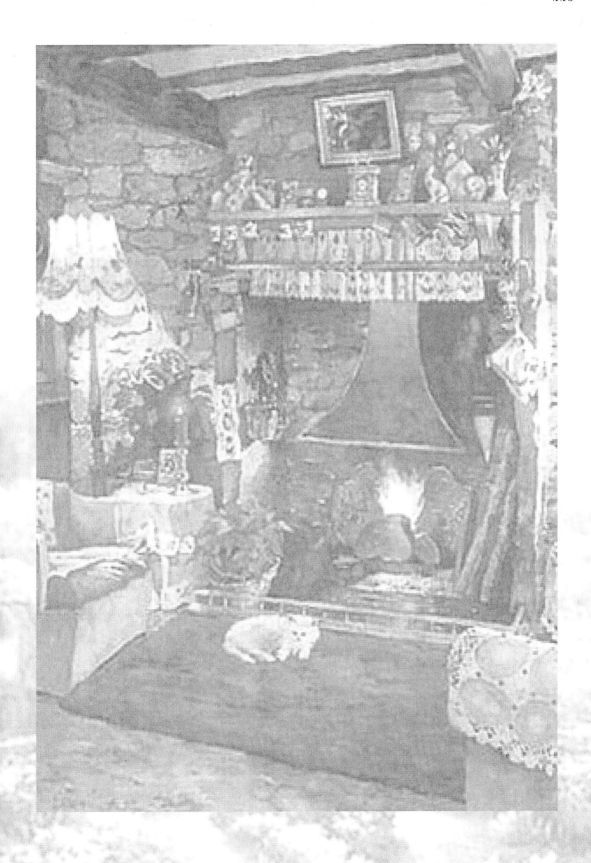

Barbie's Banana Cream Mousse

2 cups heavy cream
1 pkg. sugar-free banana cream pudding
    mix (instant)
1 tsp. coconut extract

First... with mixer, beat heavy cream and banana cream pudding (instant), until smooth and creamy. Pour into margarita glasses. Top with a Coconut macaroon or two, from this book. Put in the refrigerator and chill at least an hour. Can top with some whip cream, sugar- free of course. You can make it by taking 1-1 ½ cups heavy cream and 2 tsp. Splenda and whipping in bowl until soft peaks form. May also add a flavoring or extract to the cream before you beat it.

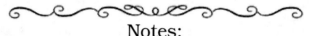

Notes:

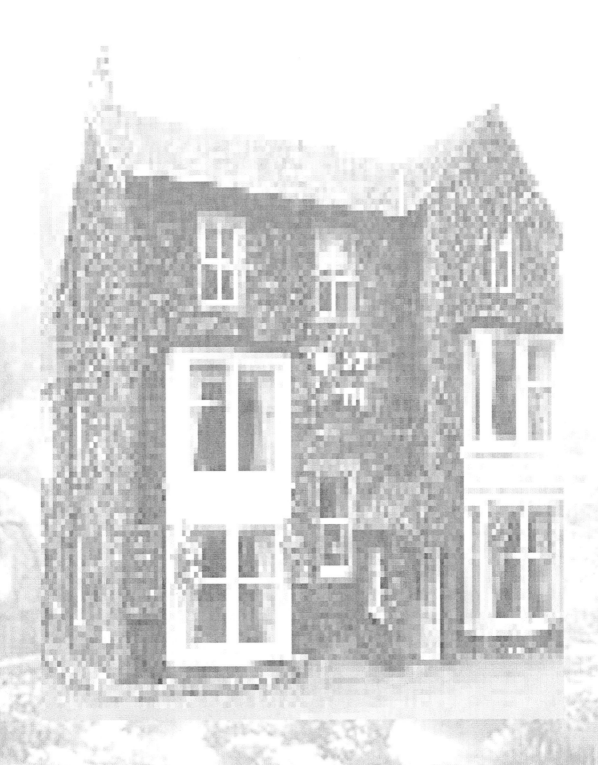

Rocco's Wild Bananas Foster

6 egg yolks
6 oz. Splenda
the peel of half an orange, with none of the white pith
1 Tbsp. Grand Marnier liqueur (Triple Sec will do)
16 oz. milk

First... put the egg yolks and sugar into a bowl and beat until it becomes pale yellow and forms soft ribbons.

Next... put the cream and orange peel in a saucepan, turn the heat to medium and bring the milk to a slow simmer. Do not let it break into a boil.

Next... add the hot milk to the beaten yolks, pouring it in a thin stream through a fine strainer. Add a little at a time, stopping after each time to beat it into the yolks. Add the Grand Marnier, stirring well.

Next... transfer the mixture to a saucepan, turn the heat to medium and beat constantly for about 2 minutes, letting it boil, then take off the heat and allow it to become completely cool.

Freezing the Gelato... pour the mixture, making sure it is already very cold, into the container of your ice cream maker and freeze it following the manufacturer's instructions. When done, the Gelato is ready to eat, but if you want to serve it later, or prefer it when it's more compact, transfer it to a container that closes tightly and place in the freezer. If you are going to leave it in the freezer overnight or longer, let the Gelato soften a little by putting it in the refrigerator for 30 minutes.

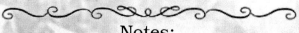

Notes:

Do you absolutely flip for Bananas Foster? You probably will when you check this one out! It takes a little effort... but let me tell you, the end result if out of this world!

Assembling the Bananas Foster

1 jar of sugar-free caramel or butterscotch topping*
3 Tbsp. butter
3 bananas, peeled and sliced diagonally
2 Tbsp. rum plus ½ tsp. rum extract
egg custard Gelato
½ tsp. lemon zest, grated

First... melt butter in skillet and add bananas and lemon zest. Sauté bananas until they become caramelized.

Next... add one cup of the caramel or butterscotch sugar-free topping, ½ tsp. rum extract and simmer until heated through. Add rum and flambé!

Serving suggestion: Take martini or margarita glasses and scoop the egg custard Gelato into the glass. Top with flaming banana caramel mixture.

My guess is that if you do not go gaga on the bananas, one serving is less than 10 carbs. Still a much better substitute than that normal hot fudge sundae. All is good!

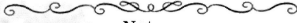

Notes:
Smuckers carries a sugar-free caramel and chocolate topping

TIP: you can substitute sugar free ice-cream from the store for the Gelato and that's ok! But the flavor and texture will never be the same. There is also a sugar-free caramel ice cream topping to follow, in case you can't find one in the store.

Sugar-Free Butterscotch Ice Cream Topping

1 cup Splenda
½ cup water
1 ½ cups heavy cream
3 Tbsp. butter

Combine sugar and water in medium pan. (add water a Tbsp. at a time). Cook over high heat until mixture is a light golden brown. Remove from heat and add cream and stir until smooth. Cool the sauce and top your ice cream. Leftovers can be re-heated.

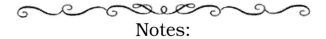

Notes:

Sugar-Free Hot fudge Ice Cream Topping

4 (1oz.) squares of unsweetened chocolate
½ cup butter
½ tsp. salt
3 cups Splenda
1 can (12 oz.) evaporated milk

First... fill the lower pot of a double boiler half way and bring to a boil. Melt chocolate, butter and salt together in upper pot. Add the sugar, ½ cup at a time, stirring after each addition.

Next... gradually add the evaporated milk, a little at a time and continue stirring until well mixed. Serve hot over ice cream. Extra sauce may be stored in refrigerator and re hated in microwave.

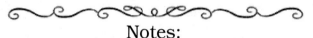

Notes:

A TIME TO REFLECT

Friends, in all seriousness, we have come to a point in the book in which we should take a moment to reflect upon ourselves. How do we feel about ourselves? How do feel about food? How do we feel about the amount of food we eat at a particular meal? How many times do we eat when we are not really hungry? Are we just eating to amuse ourselves? How many times do we turn to food to cover up our hurt, pain, humiliation, and exhaustion? How about loneliness, sadness, depression, guilt or despair?... Anger, boredom, irritability and even bereavement? Next time you put food in your mouth, kindly ask yourself, "Am I doing it for any of these reasons?" Are you really waiting for that hunger pang in your stomach to let you know it is ready to re-fuel again? The equation is simple. If you put food into your stomach before you have used up the last supply of food, you are going to put more food into your body than you need, ergo, you are going to gain weight. If you only eat when you are really, really hungry and wait for that to burn off, (no matter how many hours it takes to burn it off) even if you have to miss the following meal, you are not going to have a weight problem. (Assuming that you will apply this principle once you have reached your goal weight). Learn to listen to your body! It will tell you when it is really hungry. God created the perfect system. The problem is... we do not listen.

If you are a human being, you were born with a "soul connection" to your Creator. This is a Truth that is and will remain in existence whether you choose to believe it or not. If the "soul connection" to our Creator is not turned on, or it is neglected, willfully or not, you will experience a void in your life, a void that never seems to go away. Some experience this as unexplained depression, loneliness, sadness, anxiety, uneasiness, unhappiness and a host of other negative feelings. This happens because your Creator is "Light" and if you are not connected to the "Light", you remain connected to the "dark". When you are connected to the "dark", you only experience what the "dark" has to offer you. Hence forth, you are constantly in search of something you can not find. You search and you search for love, laughter and true joy from within and yet you can never seem to find it. This is the very thing that leaves you with all of those dark feelings and voids. You don't know what to do, and so the next best thing that you have found to do is called "comfort eating". This is great! Comforting! However, it is only a temporary fix, which in the long run leaves you feeling worse than ever. Sensations of guilt, disgust, despair and frustration... even desperation usually lie at the bottom of all of this, thus creating an even larger problem.

There are two kinds of food. "Soul Food" and "Body Food". When you learn how to feed the soul, the body will take care of it's own. I really believe that the reason we eat so much is that we think we are feeding our hungry stomachs when what we are really trying to fill are the deep hungers and desires of the soul. My friends, there are no earthly foods that can feed the cries of the soul. We eat and eat to feel better, yet we never seem full... And we keep paying for it over and over with excess body weight. The answer is simple... feed the soul! Consume your soul with the wonderment of the Heavenly Father, the One who loves you so much that He gave His only begotten son so that you may never perish, but have everlasting life! Do you think that the One who gave His only begotten Son for you, would not be there to help you in your struggles? When you become consumed with Him instead of food, you will see the light! Seek and you shall find! Ask and you shall receive! Knock and the door will be opened! Experience for yourself, the light of your Heavenly Father and all the blessings it brings to you. Your Father in Heaven EXISTS to love you, share with you, and bless you in more ways than you could ever imagine, but He can't do it unless you ask Him to do it.

Fill your hunger with the "Bread of Life"... not the emptiness of obesity!

Your loving Father did not create you to be unhappy, lonely, empty, over weight and oppressed. He created you to have an abundant, joyful and prosperous life! He created you to bless you all the days of your life, another Truth that did, does and will continue to exist whether you believe it or not. So why not believe it and receive it? Remember, receiving is in direct proportion to believing! Ultimately, our Heavenly Father does have... The last Dance!

Yes, we talk about celebrating life, family, friends and food in this book because life should be celebrated to the fullest. However, there are ways to celebrate food to the fullest without consuming quantities to the fullest. I am convinced that celebrating food to the fullest can mean enjoying the flavor, uniqueness of the recipe, presentation of the food, the people you are sharing the dining experience with and even the smells that fill the air. It doesn't have to be all about the quantity, and eating until you drop over and can't move. Whether it is carbohydrates or proteins we are talking about, there is nothing comforting about stretching out your stomach just to get the feeling of fullness. That stretched out stomach just requires more food to fill it. Our goal in this book is to try to get you to start enjoying the quality of the food instead of the quantity. It's about filling all the senses, not all of the stomach. Our guess is that if you start enjoying every aspect of the meal, this will fill you up, not the quantity of the food you consume. We need to start acknowledging the fact there WILL be more food available to us after the meal we are currently eating and if we feel the need to leave some of it on our plate this time around, just do it! So many of us have a hard time leaving food on our plate! One reason of course being the age we grew up in and the guilt trip about those "starving children". We need to get rid of that line of thinking right now. If we finish all the food on our plate, it certainly isn't going to help the "starving children" anyway. If you want to help the "starving children", eat less and send money. Although it may sound funny, you wouldn't believe how many people tell me that this was pounded into their head as a child and stuck with them all through their life. Check out the program in your head! What got you to the point you are at in life? All programs can be re-programmed!

The beauty of this book is that we are all struggling along together. We all know what to do, we just have a hard time doing it. Or, we don't know how to do it at all. We are in the same boat as you are. We are not trying to give you unrealistic goals to reach as we sit here in our bikinis weighing in at 115 pounds. I can assure you that we are a support group of friends with the same problems that surround you daily. We have the same feelings, the same joys the same sorrows, and the same concerns. We are one as a family so let's come together and share some little steps that will help us become the people we want to be!

GIVING THANKS

Friends, in leaving you now, I would like to use this opportunity to thank you for taking the time to look at this book.

Were we able to help you in your struggle to stay on track?

I sincerely hope that the recipes we shared with you will help you make some changes that will stay with you a lifetime.

This book was a labor of love to all of my friends who suffer as I do with this addiction. A lot of these things have helped me. I was hoping to pass them on to you, so that your lives may become a little more enjoyable, and I hope we got to know each other a little along the way!

The perspective of this book may have been a little bold, but it was "pure" in the sense that we need to know that there are people out there who ARE just like us. We are real people with real feelings, living in a very real world. A world that places entirely too much emphasis on the most beautiful of faces, the sexiest of bodies and the biggest and best of material possessions. We can all strive to be better people, but friends... Let's love ourselves along the way. Let's get the biggest kick out of life that we can! Let's have the most fun we can at it and enjoy everything around us! Life may pass you by before you make it to the "Sports Illustrated, Swim Suit Edition". The "perfect" body does not always get you the perfect mate, the best job, the most beautiful home and in fact, it can't even buy you happiness. Happiness comes from within my friends and only you can make that happen! Be thin to be healthy, that is a good thing, but you are already a BEAUTIFUL person in who you are! Start living for today... because you just don't know what tomorrow will bring!

Cover art by Kay Miland
Editing and design by William Wilson

Note for Librarians: a cataloguing record for this book that includes Dewey Classification and US Library of Congress numbers is available from the National Library of Canada. The complete cataloguing record can be obtained from the National Library's online database at: www.nlc-bnc.ca/amicus/index-e.html

ISBN 1-4120-3101-X

TRAFFORD

This book was published on-demand in cooperation with Trafford Publishing. On-demand publishing is a unique process and service of making a book available for retail sale to the public taking advantage of on-demand manufacturing and Internet marketing. On-demand publishing includes promotions, retail sales, manufacturing, order fulfilment, accounting and collecting royalties on behalf of the author.

Suite 6E, 2333 Government St., Victoria, B.C. V8T 4P4, CANADA
Phone   250-383-6864   Toll-free 1-888-232-4444 (Canada & US)
Fax   250-383-6804   E-mail   sales@trafford.com
Web site www.trafford.com TRAFFORD PUBLISHING IS A DIVISION OF TRAFFORD HOLDINGS LTD.
Trafford Catalogue #04-0928   www.trafford.com/robots/04-0928.html

10   9   8   7   6   5   4   3   2   1

ISBN 141203101-X